My Nights
with
Leukemia

My Nights
with
Leukemia

Caring for Children
with Cancer

Michael W. Perry

Inkling Books   Auburn   2013

Description

A moving and realistic look at what it was like to care for children with cancer, particularly leukemia, on night shift in the Hematology-Oncology unit at one of the nation's top children's hospitals.

Copyright Notice

Dedication

To all the children I cared for and their families.

Library Cataloging Data

Title: *My Nights with Leukemia: Caring for Children with Cancer*
Author: Michael W. Perry (1948–).

Description:

204 pages and 50 pictures, including stock photos from Big Stock Photos and Deposit Photos, used with permission.
Size: 6 x 9 x 0.5 inches, 229 x 152 x 12 mm. Weight: 0.7 pounds, 310 grams.
Library of Congress Control Number: 2013911739 (paper edition).
BISAC Subject Headings:
MED058050   MEDICAL / NURSING / FUNDAMENTALS & SKILLS
MED058160   MEDICAL / NURSING / ONCOLOGY & CANCER
MED058080   MEDICAL / NURSING / PEDIATRIC & NEONATAL
MED069000   MEDICAL / PEDIATRICS
MED062000   MEDICAL / ONCOLOGY
ISBN for paperback: 978-1-58742-074-0
ISBN for ePub: 978-1-58742-075-7 (iBookstore)
ISBN for Kindle: 978-1-58742-076-4 (Amazon)
ISBN for Smashwords: 978-1-58742-077-1 (Other digital editions)

Publisher Information

Print edition published in the United States of America on acid-free paper.
First edition. First printing
Publisher: Inkling Books, Auburn, AL, August 2013.
Internet: http://www.InklingBooks.com/

CONTENTS

1. AN UNUSUAL PATH

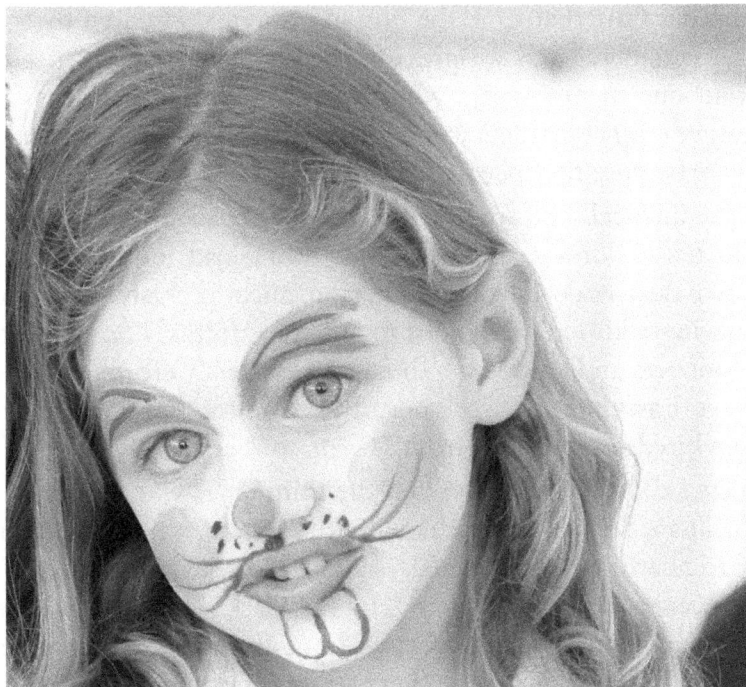

The path that led me to working nights caring for children with leukemia was an unusual one. Working as the director of a group home for drug addicts led to stresses that I thought were best relieved by a different stress—mountain climbing. Almost getting killed several times while climbing in turn led me to take an Emergency Medical Technician course at a local community college. If I or a fellow climber were badly injured far from assistance, I wanted to know what to do.

Just after finishing that EMT course, a friend from church mentioned that she'd applied for a pediatric aide position at a nearby children's hospital and that I might want to apply too. "Interesting," I thought, "that'd let me use that EMT training." Interesting proved an understatement.

At that time, EMT training easily qualified me for the position. Aide work was hands-on patient care, meaning diaper changes for the younger kids, bedsheets for everyone, trays of food at meal times, and the like. That's what nursing assistants do in hospitals today. As I began, it seemed the only part of the job that was medical was taking a child's vital signs—typically heart rate, respiration, and temperature—every four hours. My training appeared more than enough.

A week of classroom training was followed by three weeks of orientation on days. At that time the hospital assigned children by age and type of treatment. I was assigned to the medical unit, which handled kids from one to nine years who typically received medicines rather than surgery. Since parents can usually handle pills, many of our kids were there because they needed an IV.

On the medical unit, we had three clusters of rooms, each with from seven to ten children—about the right work load for a nurse and an aide. Two clusters dealt with ordinary medical problems, with one of those having additional isolation rooms for infections or, as we called them, "poopers and croopers." Those two clusters were where I trained and where I assumed I'd work once I took up the position for which I had been hired, a night shift from 11 p.m. to 7 a.m.

I knew I didn't want to work on the third or "A Cluster," as we then called it. It specialized in treating children from birth to nine with cancers, particularly leukemia, which is a cancer of the blood and the most common cancer among children. Because Alaska and three other states were served by our hospital, children from almost one-fourth the land mass of the United States came there for treatment.

Later, that seven-room cluster took over the space for the entire medical unit and became a specialized wing of the hospital that's called Hem-Onc, from *Hem*atology (diseases of the blood) and *Onc*ology (cancers). Since the term is short and clear, I'll use Hem-Onc to describe those special rooms for children with cancers. Currently, the hospital ranks among the top-ten children's hospitals in the country and offers some of the best care in the world for children with leukemia.

I can easily explain why I didn't want to work Hem-Onc. First, look at the picture of the lovely little girl at the start of this chapter (as well as the front cover of the print edition). Made up to look like a bunny, perhaps for a birthday party, she seems in robust good health, doesn't she? Now look at the girl whose picture opens the next chapter (and the back cover of the print edition). Yes, it's the same girl, maybe only a few months later. She's been diagnosed with leukemia and blasted with the horrors of chemotherapy.

Those two pictures demonstrate far better than any words I might say what working on Hem-Onc meant. It meant being one of those who transformed children who came in looking like the first picture into those who looked like the second. Would you want to do that? Neither did I. There was nothing I wanted less to do. Nothing at all.

Today, children like her are kept in isolated units to reduce still further the chance of an infection, but that wasn't true then. I could see patients like her as I hurried about just yards away on B Cluster. They looked like the survivors of a terrible concentration camp or the victims of some demented medical sadism. They were pale and thin, with only a few wisps of hair on bald heads. They walked haltingly, often with a parent or nurse alongside pushing a pole loaded with several IV pumps and bags. It was grim, grim, grim.

There was no danger, I reminded myself, that I would ever work there. While the hospital as a whole practiced 'team nursing,' matching a nurse with an aide like me, the cancer unit had kids who were much sicker and was, so I believed, all-nurse. Also, the risk of spreading an infection to children who had little or no immune system was so great, staff not specifically assigned there rarely came near its patients. It was a world unto itself—a terrifying world I had no desire to join.

Then my month-long orientation ended, and I arrived for my first night shift. It was then that I discovered I'd been specifically hired to work with those kids battling cancer. It was true—I now found out—that on day shift, only nurses worked Hem-Onc. But on night shift it was staffed with a nurse and an aide. I was to be that aide.

Later, the hospital's head of nursing told me why I'd been given that assignment. Knowing that these kids were extremely sick, literally at death's door, they needed to two highly qualified aides to alternate filling that single slot each night of the week. The already-filled position was held by a talented third-year nursing student. My EMT training had won me the second position. With no medical background other than those EMT classes—two nights a week of emergency medicine for three months—I'd been assigned one of the most demanding aide positions in a top-tier children's hospital.

On that first night, I wondered what I was in for. Could I manage to cope with something I'd wanted to avoid at all costs? Would I be willing to pay the heavy emotional cost of caring for terribly sick and often dying children? Most important of all, could I learn to give these children the medical care they so desperately needed?

2. Accepting the Challenge

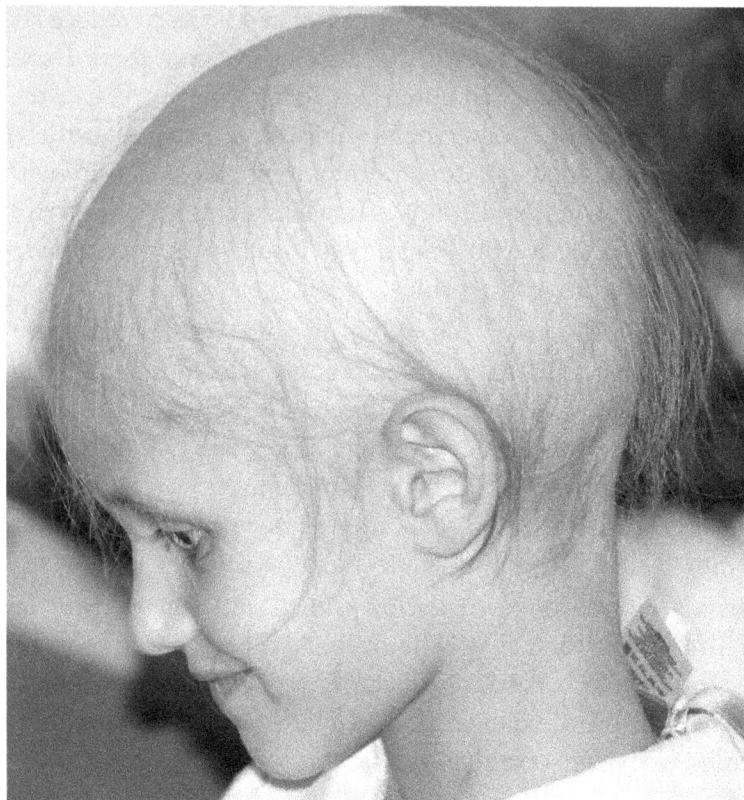

Discovering that I was to work nights on Hem-Onc was one of the most unsettling experiences of my life. After a month of training in caring for kids who weren't that sick, I suddenly found myself expected to care for children who were battling cancers that could easily kill them—terribly sick kids that I'd not wanted to get near just days before

How did I make the transition? To be honest, I don't know. It happened so quickly, I don't recall the details. One moment I was shocked to discover that I was to do the very work I'd wanted to avoid at all costs. The next, my memories are of wanting to work with these kids to the exclusion of all else. It may have taken several hours. It may have taken several nights. I'm not sure. All I know is that it happened quickly.

What I do remember was that my attitude changed so completely, I soon clashed with the nursing student who shared that Hem-Onc slot. Three nights a week—Wednesday, Thursday, and Friday—we were both on duty. She felt as strongly as I did about caring for those children, so we had to reach an agreement that, when Wednesday came around, whoever had been caring for those kids would continue to do so until their two-day break came. Then the other half of our dynamic duo took over. That gave those kids continuity of care. When she was caring for them, she knew the most about their circumstances. A few days later when I took over, I'd have picked up from her what I needed to know.

A little background will help you understand our work schedule. For staffing, the hospital alternated three days on and two off with seven on and two off. Odd as a 7/3 rotation sounds—too many days on alternating with too few—it has one big advantage. It gave nursing staff every other weekend off. Weekends off made our lives a bit more normal.

My surprising change of mind suggests three insights that you might remember, especially if you're planning on a career in medicine, nursing, or any other demanding profession. In fact, these insights should be helpful whenever life brings great difficulties your way.

The first insight is that doing something is radically different from merely observing it. Working on Hem-Onc proved utterly unlike seeing it from a mere thirty feet away. Fear does not survive liking. Those frail figures who had so terrified me when they were strangers, quickly became children I knew and loved. That's one reason why a direct experience affects us far more deeply than a book, a film, or what we see as visitors merely passing through.

I saw that while mountain climbing. A real climb, I discovered, is never like watching a movie or driving past a mountain. After what I called my Summer of Living Dangerously, books and films about climbing were never the same. They fell into two groups. The best captured a small slice of the reality. The worst were useless.

That even the best films can only capture a slice of powerful experiences comes from our human limitations as chroniclers along with the limited span of any media. Mountain climbing is beautiful almost beyond belief. There's nothing that compares to being able to see, on a clear day, a hundred miles or more in every direction. Being on a mountain can also be eerie and mysterious, particularly on a glacier at night, when all sense of distance and perspective disappear, leaving everything strange and other-worldly.

It's also brutal and exhausting. In my case, climbing Mount Rainier nonstop—something only macho climbers attempt—meant being awake for some 32 hours and constantly on the move for nearly 24 hours. When a Japanese exchange student seemed to think that climbing it would be like topping Japan's cute Mt. Fuji, I was blunt. Pick one of Seattle's taller skyscrapers, I told her, and go up and down its 600-feet of stairs sixteen times with a forty-pound pack without resting. That, roughly put, that's what summiting the 14,411-foot Mt. Rainier is like. It's a grind—a long miserable grind.

I experienced that grind and hated it. Coming down from Mt. Rainier, I was so tired I told myself that I never wanted to see another mountain again, much less climb one. Alas, two weeks later I was making an attempt on the 11,138-foot Little Tahoma, which is a side peak to Mt. Rainier. On that climb, we had to cross a portion of glacier so filled with crevasses, my fellow climber and I took two hours to travel a mere quarter of a mile. That was how dangerous it was. At times we could see three crevasses in the 50-feet of rope that separated us. I even fell into an hidden one, wedging up to my waist in the snow. It was so frustrating, I could only cope by laughing.

Those changing attitude, for, against, and then for, illustrates that climbing has benefits and costs. The grind, terrible as it is, makes you strong-willed and teaches you to deal with being tired and yet go on because you must. You'll never acquire that sitting on a couch watching a mountaineering movie. That 'do it because you must' experience mattered when I faced those long nights on Hem-Onc, when I dare not let myself get sleepy.

Finally, to all those varied feelings add the omnipresence of danger. In the midst of beauty, mystery, and exhaustion, mountain climbing is also deadly. At any moment you may be called on to respond correctly in an instant or die. That happened three times during my Summer of Living Dangerously. Each time—and with no advanced warning—I had from a split second to a couple of seconds to react properly or see either myself or a fellow climber die. That too was like Hem-Onc, where the lives of our children depended on the decisions I made.

A talented movie director may be able to capture one or two of those realities, but not all and certainly not all at the same time. Yet that simultaneity is how I experienced it. Not just beauty and then death, but beauty alongside death. The two are one and the same.

That simultaneity was particularly vivid for me when I saved another climber from a nasty fall on Mount Constance, a large peak in the

Olympic Mountains just across Puget Sound from Seattle. We were roped together and, had I failed in my arrest, that evening would have found both of us badly injured and looking across the waters at the lovely lights of Seattle twinkling in the distance—beauty in the midst of death.

Working Hem-Onc was similar. Alongside danger and death, there was beauty and a unique experience of life's joys. I vividly recall one morning when I finished my usual end-of-shift tasks early. With no demands on my time, one of my little patients and I went to a small play area, where she proceeded to rip pages out of magazines, looking to me for reassurance that what she was doing was OK.

That was a special moment. Earlier, doctors had given this little girl almost no chance of leaving the ICU alive. Even now, transferred to Hem-Onc, she faced a desperate battle with a rare form of leukemia, Yet for those few stolen moments, the two of us could enjoy being together as a lovely early morning sun streamed in through the windows. And fortunately, I had my camera with me that morning. Those moments are captured forever in the pictures that accompany the chapters about her. Here, I'll call her Jackie. In real life she has another name.

C. S. Lewis expressed much the same feeling about death in *A Grief Observed* when he described his last days and hours with his much-loved wife: "It is incredible how much happiness, even how much gaiety, we sometimes had together after all hope was gone. How long, how tranquilly, how nourishingly, we talked together that last night!"

Experiences like those are why caring for desperately sick and often dying children proved such a revelation. Today, when I tell friends about what I did then, they usually become shocked, and wonder how anyone could do that. "No," I feel like screaming. "It wasn't what you think. If you'd been in my situation, you'd have probably felt like I did. I wanted to work there. I didn't want to do anything else."

How can I explain that? Here's a feeble attempt. Recently I read of a study that explored why couples raise children. It's exhausting, and it's expensive. It can often be painful. Why don't they avoid kids and live only for themselves? The researchers concluded that those very burdens are what made parenthood attractive. Because it was hard, doing it well gave a sense of accomplishment that childless couples never experience.

Working with kids battling leukemia and other cancers was like that. Caring for them exacted a heavy toll. The work was hard, sometimes unpleasant, and always stressful. Every night when I came to work, I knew that one slip on my part might cost a child's life. Every night, tired or not, I reminded myself to do my best. On top of that, it was painful when a child that I cared about died after a months-long battle—although nothing like the pain the child's parents felt.

But along with that suffering came a sense of accomplishment. Modern medicine is enormously powerful. On the other two clusters of the medical unit, there was little doubt that almost every kid would get well and go home. We were simply making their sickness more comfortable and briefer.

But with the kids on Hem-Onc, I could make a life or death difference. Around the clock, these children's lives hung in the balance. Death could come suddenly. On Monday, one little boy I was caring for was happy, alert and medically stable. On Wednesday he died in the ICU from an out-of-control infection. On another morning about 5 a.m. a boy told me his head hurt. A half-hour later, as the code team rushed him to the ICU, I knew there was no hope. He was dying of a massive brain hemorrhage. That was the reality I faced each and every night. The lives of our children often hung by the thinnest of threads. There I made a difference, and that's why the work was so special. You may find what you do special too, so don't fear a challenge like that.

The second insight was the realization that we can cope with challenges far better than we imagine. Our power to adapt to new situations is often far greater than we realize. That's why I get angry at those who say, "I couldn't do that." Many could. Necessity really can change us. We can become what we must be. Actions that seem impossible from a distance may prove doable up close. As a story I read in high school put it, "a boy becomes a man when a man is needed." Need can make us what we must be.

That's also true of life in general. One aspect of my short craze for mountain climbing still amazes me. I have few phobias, but one of them is heights. Place me on top of a building looking down over a parapet, and I get tense and nervous, even though falling is impossible. Yet put me on a mountain and place me on a narrow ledge, with a fatal fall mere inches away, and I become cool, calm, and collected. I can look down without flinching by simply telling myself that I must stay oriented.

No, I don't fully understand why that's true. As best I can tell, it has to do with purpose and necessity. I have *purposed* to climb that peak, so

My Nights with Leukemia

anything *necessary* for that must be embraced. Fear of heights is out of place on a mountain, so that fear must go. To do what I must do, I must accept what I cannot change.

That's also true in the messier corners of medicine. We often find that we *can* do what we *must* do. Recall nineteenth-century Victorian England, where women from the more affluent classes were kept away from anything unsightly or stressful. They were pampered and treated as helpless children. Some felt it was ladylike to faint at the sight of a tiny drop of blood. Yet some of those same women, serving as nurses with Florence Nightingale in the Crimean War, proved strong, courageous, and resourceful. Surrounded by blood, gore and death, they remained calm, caring, and professional.

A new situation can work like that. It can transform us and bring out strengths we never knew we had. And yes, not everyone has that strength, but many do. You'll never know until you try. So don't say no to a challenge, even when it comes unbidden and unwanted, as it did that first night when I found I was assigned to Hem-Onc.

That same transforming power of adversity was also true of many children with cancer. One example is the lovely girl whose photos you see on the cover and at the start of the first three chapters as well as elsewhere in this book. I don't know her name, so I'll refer to her simply as The Girl.

Her professionally done pictures didn't begin with her leukemia. Her father or mother must be a photographer. Online, she has stock photos that go back to when she was about three years old. The one at the start of the first chapter was probably taken when she was about eight and just before her leukemia was diagnosed. That at the start of this chapter was taken at the height of her chemotherapy and that at the start of the next chapter was probably made when she was in remission and recovering. Notice her hair is coming back.

It's easy to imagine that, when her treatment began, her parents asked her if she wanted to continue to have her pictures taken—stock photos of children with leukemia being very rare. In response, she must have said, "Yes, I want to do it because it might help other children who're going through what I'm going through."

That illustrates what it was often like to care for these children. Sometimes they amazed me. Often, I felt privileged to care for them. In every case, it was nothing like what I'd imagined from a distance.

The third insight came when I realized that what happened to me mattered little. I'll write more on that later, but for now keep in mind that, surrounded by so much suffering and death, the petty issues and difficulties in my own life shrank into insignificance. I wasn't enduring the horrors of chemotherapy. I wasn't facing a serious possibility of dying, and even if I were, I could face dying as an adult rather than as a frightened little child. There was, I soon discovered, something wrong with thinking much about myself. I had work to do that mattered more than any passing mood of my own.

That 'not me' attitude proved especially critical when I first began working Hem-Onc. Recall that I had been trained in outside-the-hospital emergency medicine. I was far better prepared to deliver unexpected babies than to treat a baby with cancer. Even my three weeks of formal orientation had not prepared me. I had trained for the ordinary sicknesses of a medical unit. Only much later did I realize that the failure of the unit's head nurse to assign at least part of my orientation period to Hem-Onc was an early warning of trouble to come. Until I reported to work nights, I was taught nothing about leukemia care.

Knowing virtually nothing about the intricacies of treating cancer, in desperation I turned to the other meaning of the word care. Failure, I promised myself, would not result from any lack of effort. Come what may, I'd love my young patients and do my very best for them. During those first few weeks, as I struggled to learn my job, that love was all I had to offer. I couldn't use my knowledge, training or experience, because I had none. Fortunately, that proved enough.

That, in a nutshell, is the special world I'll be describing in this book. I will be telling you what it was like to spend nights with children who were dying or almost certainly could die. I will be showing you a world in which suffering and death came mixed with beauty and a special humanity. It was a world in which I found I could do things I never thought possible.

I hope this book will inspire you to do something similar with your life. Perhaps it will help you cope with a tragedy or illness you cannot avoid. Perhaps it will motivate you to accept the challenges that come your way and to believe that you *can* do what you *must* do.

Next, we'll step back and look at one of medicine's best-kept secrets. It offers a key to understanding where I found myself during those first nights caring for children with leukemia.

3. A Secret about Nights

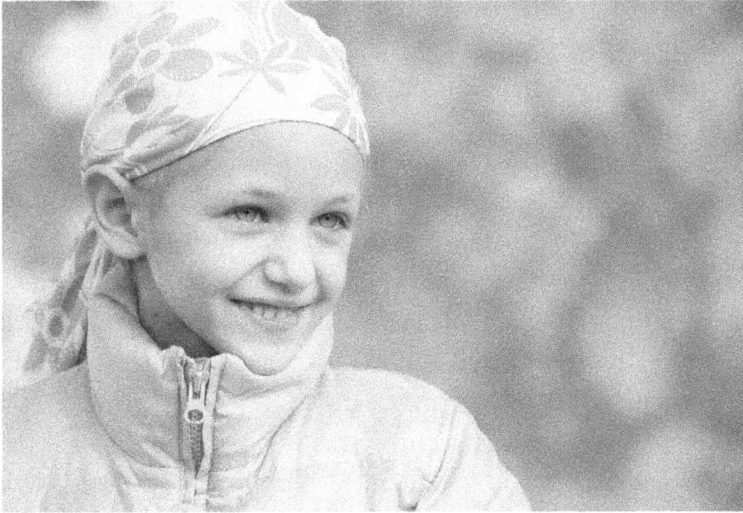

I'll let you in on a little secret—one that's more than a little scary. Hospitals have problems staffing night shifts, and it's easy to see why. We're day creatures, tuned to the rhythms of the sun. Our bodies cope poorly with being awake at night. Working nights for months on end wears you down. I know it did me.

It also wreaks havoc with your social life. Forget conversations. You're asleep when friends are awake and awake when they're asleep. They quickly develop a fear of calling at the wrong time and don't call at all. The overlap in the evening doesn't help. Go out with friends, and you spoil their fun by fretting about the time when you must leave. As bad as night shifts are for singles, they're still worse for those with a spouse and kids. A marriage can become like two ships passing in the night. Without planning, a couple will spend little time together.

As a result, at many hospitals the night shifts are an anti-fringe benefit imposed on the newly hired. People grudgingly take nights to get a job. Once they build up seniority, they look for an opening on day or evening shift. I saw that happen many times.

Unfortunately, that start-on-nights policy often means that night shifts have the least experienced staff. Still worse is the fact that a hospital's staff count is also down in the middle of the night, when sensible people are in bed and there are few experienced physicians on duty.

That's particularly true at teaching hospitals, where nights are typically covered by residents, doctors-in-training who may have no more that a few weeks experience with a particular kind of care. When a crisis develops, a nurse, who may be fresh out of nursing school, faces a terrible dilemma: "It's 3 a.m. Do I call a resident who knows even less than I do, or do I wake up the attending physician who's never heard my name?" Not an easy choice.

I still remember when I called the resident on duty one night about Ralph, the name I've given a boy of about eight who had complained to me of a headache. The instant I finished explaining, she said, "I'm calling the attending, then I'll be right down." Hearing that, I realized this boy was in serious trouble. At our hospital, the attending physician was often a nationally recognized specialist thus a Very Important Person. Residents only woke them for a very good reason.

In Ralph case, there was nothing she or I could do. He was doomed the moment a tiny blood vessel inside his brain popped. A normal count for the platelets that are in our blood to stop bleeding is around 300,000. At my hospital, a platelet count under 20,000 was considered a life-threatening emergency. There was a standing order that, whenever a patient's lab results dropped into that range, day or night, the medical technician was to immediately call the patient's attending physician. A count of 20,000 could kill.

Ralph's last platelet count had been 6,000, less than a third of that already life-threatening number. Normally he would have been given a platelet infusion, but he'd received so many, his body was resistant. That night we were attempting to coast him through that crisis. Unfortunately, we failed. In the end, it's hard to know how we could have done otherwise. Some situations have no easy answers.

In other situations, the delay in calling a resident, the resident arriving to make an assessment, and then the specialist being called and becoming involved can be fatal. During the day, top-notch skill is only a few minutes away. At night it can take two hours or more to arrive.

Other factors also matter. If I were a doctor, I'd never want to make decisions from far away and only seconds after being awakened from a deep sleep. Yet that's what they must do. All that is to say that nights are not a good time to find yourself in a medical crisis. Yet there I was, new to medicine and working nights caring for some of the sickest kids in a top-tier hospital.

Finally, there's ample evidence—anecdotal and statistical—that medical crises are more likely to develop during the wee hours of the night as our bodies slow down during deep sleep. I never collected actual data, but it did seem that while I was on night shift—one third of each day—we had half or more of the medical emergencies and deaths.

The only saving grace was that, while a problem may have begun around three or four a.m., it often did not surface until after five a.m., and the more ample staffing and expertise of day shift began arriving about six a.m. By the time we knew we needed help, it was often arriving, much like the calvary riding over the hill in an old-time western. That could be a blessed relief.

Next, we look at my introduction to night shift, and the crucial role my first nurses played.

4. Learning from Nurses

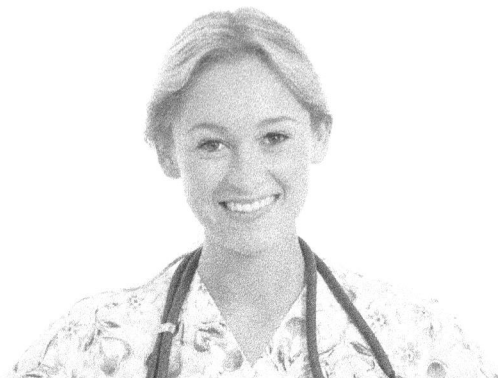

Fortunately for me, the usual pattern that night nursing staff were less skilled wasn't true. All the nurses I began working with were experienced both at nursing in general and on Hem-Onc in particular. They would teach me well.

First, from them I learned the importance of staying on the move, making my rounds and continually looking in on the kids. Technically, I was seeing if they had any obvious needs, such as a diaper change or a drink of water, but I was also watching for problems.

That was especially important with the age of patients we had. Most teens, I later discovered, won't hesitate to complain. But childhood leukemia peaks about age four and most cases are between two and eight. Kids that young aren't good at telling strange adults what's happening to them, so it's important to move constantly between their rooms.

The same rule applies to parents. After a couple of months in a hospital, parents of seriously ill children become good at spotting problems and making sure their child gets attention. But new parents are often too intimidated to hit a call button. Coming into the room gives them a chance to speak up. So round and round I went all through the night.

Second, I learned the importance of recording everything immediately. It's hard enough to remember something during the day. In the strange and ethereal 'Twilight Zone' that's a hospital at night, there are few aids to memory. The unit is isolated. With the halls lit, but the rooms in darkness, it's a world unto itself. No one comes or goes. The awake world is only a nurse and me making our rounds. Because it's dark outside, there are no clues to the time. Even allotted breaks help little. I never took coffee breaks. There wasn't enough time. It was hard enough to find time for a middle-of-the-night equivalent of lunch, so my free moments were unpredictable. I learned that, if it happens, write it down. Otherwise, I might forget something that mattered.

Third, I discovered the importance of keeping a running to-do list. Leukemia patients typically have suppressed immune systems, making them prone to infections that appear as temperature spikes of several degrees. Those infections can kill. When their temperature first rises, the usual procedure was to take a sample of blood for culture and sensitivity (C&S) testing. The *culture* establishes what organism is causing the infection. The *sensitivity* determines which antibiotics will work against it. After that blood draw, a child was given Tylenol to lower his temperature and make him more comfortable.

My responsibilities included catching that initial temperature spike and following up the Tylenol with another temperature check an hour later. With so much to do and so little time, it was easy to forget that second check. So when a nurse made it clear to me that I could not miss those checks, I did a sensible thing. I got a small pocket alarm and set it to go off at the proper time. I learned that, if you make a mistake, it does no good to just berate yourself. Come up with a fix that keeps it from happening again. That was an important lesson.

Fourth, from a stricter-than-average nurse, I learned that even kindness can be misplaced. It's important not skip something that matters simply because it upsets a sick child. She believed that, "every kid will pee on my shift." In vain did I point out that a particular patient was a nine-year-old boy, that he was in remission, that he had no IV running, and that his chemotherapy had not yet started. He was, I plead with her, in no different a situation than when he was at home the night before, when no one cared if he peed before the six a.m. or not. None of that moved her. That poor kid had to be awakened and pee, which meant I had to do it. Grrr!

In the end, I didn't adopt her "Peeing is mandatory" policy. That was a bit much. But I did learn to force kids, even very sick kids, to do things they hated because that was best for them. We were running a hospital for the sick, I reminded myself, not a cruise ship for newly weds. To deal with my frustration, I often told nurses, "A hospital is the worst place to be when you're sick." It was the worst from the standpoint of comfort and simply being left alone. Our kids were too sick to be left alone.

That necessity meant there were parts of my job that I hated. Pain, which typically meant holding a small child so an IV could be started or a blood draw made, was among the worst. Fortunately, I did so much else that was good for these children that none seemed to hold that against me. They quickly went back to sleep.

Worse than those a few seconds of pain was the prolonged discomfort and nausea our chemotherapy drugs created. In frustration at being able to do nothing else, I stayed with them, holding a bucket and assuring them that it would pass. Endured once, kids often asked to be drugged into oblivion for later rounds of chemotherapy.

The need to irritate and bother also frustrated me. The most telling example was a chemotherapy drug-from-hell called cisplatin. Even today, thinking about it sends my blood pressure soaring. I hate it like I hate few other things. The list of "severe side effects" at Drugs.com is chilling. The one we were most concerned about was "renal toxicity," which can occur in "25% to 36% of patients" even after a single dose. The solution was to run their IVs very fast and make them to void every two hours to flush their bladder. Later, I'd take care of a twelve-year-old boy where that hadn't been done. Every time he voided, his urine would be filled with quarter-sized blood clots. Better middle-of-the-night wake ups than that, I would tell myself.

There was, however, a problem with all that voiding. It's not normal for most kids to pee in the middle of the night, much less every two hours on demand. The result was a cruel game. The midnight void would go fine. That at two a.m. would be a bit more difficult and at four a.m. there was nothing to be had, no matter how much I urged. We'd call the resident, who'd order Lasix. It sends a strong message to kidneys saying, "Dump Urine Now!" That took care of four a.m. Unfortunately, when I came around at six a.m., Lasix had left my patient as dry as a bone. It was frustrating, but I had to try, and that poor kid had to endure my nagging. Something more important than sleep was at stake.

Pain, discomfort, and irritation at least had one redeeming aspect. As staff, we discussed them and did all we could to make them endurable. You'll read about that in this book.

Unfortunately, almost nothing was done or even discussed about one final area where a hospital stay can be unpleasant—the embarrassments and violations of privacy that are all too common. Embarrassment mattered little to the small children on Hem-Onc, but it was a major issue when I began to work day shift with teens. I soon realized that the teen guys felt under siege, well aware that the nurses caring for them were women. The same could have been true of the teen girls in my care, and I had to work hard to win their trust. I describe that experience and offer numerous suggestions about dealing with embarrassment issues in the companion volume, *Hospital Gowns and Other Embarrassments*. While the book's primary audience is teen girls, there's much that's useful for patients of any age and either sex. It's well worth reading.

Fifth, I learned from a nurse who was too relaxed to do the opposite of her. This nurse hinted a few times that I didn't really need to do all that bothersome temperature taking. All I need do, she said, was glance at a kid and, if he looked comfortable, put a made-up temperature in the charts. That made no sense, so I ignored her.

Then one night I found that one of our kids had spiked a temperature of a few degrees, a common event. When I told her, she gave me a strange look. When I went to write the boy's elevated temperature in the flow sheets, I discovered that just a few minutes before I'd taken that temperature, she'd logged a normal but obviously fake reading, perhaps to reinforce her claim that I was being too conscientious. Instead, I learned the opposite—never take anything for granted, particularly anything involving these kids. If it matters, do it.

That same nurse later became a night nurse supervisor, and I benefited from the fact that she knew I'd never be a slouch. As odd as it sounds, in her new position the nurses benefited from her more relaxed attitude. Shift supervisors need top-notch social skills, which she had. When a nurse feels overloaded and asks for additional staffing that can't be provided, she was good at calming them down. And when a night nurse needed to be persuaded stay over an additional four hours—a sleep-wrecking twelve-hour shift—she could persuade them.

That, in a nutshell, was my initial learning experience. But just as I had began to settle in, something happened that led to one of the most stressful periods I've experienced in my entire life. Hem-Onc was suddenly hit by bad news. The lives of its children would depend on how well I responded to the crisis that followed.

5. A Triple Whammy

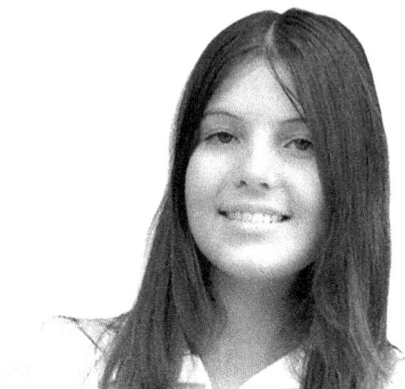

About three months after I started nights, I developed jaw pain. When I went to a friend who was a dentist, he needed only one glance in my mouth to diagnosis my problem. "Your jaw hurts because stress is causing you to grind your teeth in your sleep." He suggested I get an athletic mouth guard to deal with the grinding. Handling the stress was up to me.

I knew exactly what was causing that stress. At the hospital, I'd been hit by a triple whammy of bad news. The unthinkable had happened. Over a span of just a few weeks all the talented nurses who'd been training me left for differing reasons. Thus began the most difficult period in my care of these sick children. I would be called on to apply everything I'd learned from those nurses and more. Children's lives would depend on my woefully limited expertise.

The first bad whammy was that the experienced nurses I'd been working with all left so quickly, there was no transfer of skills to their replacements as there had been with me. Second, the nurses that replaced them were not only fresh out of nursing school, two of the three were not that capable. That might have been handled with a good orientation but for a third whammy. The nurse who handled their orientation didn't have a drill sergeant's personality, meaning she wasn't aggressive, bossy, domineering, intrusive, or whatever it took to make sure these new nurses got down pat every single move. She'd show them how to do something once and then tell them to come to her at the nurse's station if they had any problems. Not good, not good at all.

The result was sink or swim for those unfortunate nurses. During orientation, they splashed about, not knowing what they were doing, until their ignorances of the nuances and gotchas led to mistakes after their orientation was over. There were numerous mistakes, some serious.

Word spread quickly. Mothers who'd been overseeing their child's care for months and whose eagle eyes missed nothing began to lean on me. And why not? The nurses were new and blundering, while the residents were always inexperienced, typically spending only six weeks with us before rotating elsewhere. I was the only familiar, reassuring face. I was the only one not making mistakes. And I was terrified at all the responsibilities suddenly being placed on me.

Nurses on other shifts could see what was happening. Shifts start with a report time during which the nurse who's leaving explains the status of each patient to the one coming on duty. For three months, I'd been listening to a conversation between nurses. Now I got the distinct impression that the evening nurse was talking to me instead. She was expecting me to make sure nothing went wrong. Yet more tension.

One result was those grinding teeth. Remember, I'd never been to nursing school and my only medical training was that for Emergency Medical Technicians. I'd been taught how to stop bleeding wounds, splint broken bones, and deliver untimely babies. All were of little use on Hem-Onc. After only three months, I was caring for extremely sick kids in the middle of the night with no real backup. Not only must I not make mistakes of my own, I had to catch any mistakes these poorly oriented, less-than-gifted new nurses might make. It was terrible.

At this point, I should explain what I mean when I say that I found the situation terrifying. I don't mean that I was overcome with emotion or paralyzed into inaction. As I learned mountain climbing, that's not how I respond to danger. Instead, I carefully weighed the situation and found that my training and experience came up woefully lacking. It was all too easy to imagine myself failing and a child dying. Fears that flow from reasoned thought and imagination differ from those that result from an irrational, emotional reaction. I knew all too well what I feared.

For a parallel, imagine yourself walking across a meadow on a sunny day holding the hand of a small child you love. Suddenly, a lion rears up out of the thick grass only yards ahead. You have no weapon and the closest tree is so distant, you couldn't make it there running alone, much less carrying the child. What would you do?

First, you would use God's greatest gift to you—your mind—and begin to recall everything you know about dealing with lions that might help. Second, you have your hands, and—as weak as they are against sharp teeth and claws—your resolve to use them. Last but not least, you have your will. This lion will learn that he cannot get to that child without dealing with you first.

Leukemia was that lion and I responded appropriately. I ground my teeth because even as I slept my mind wrestled constantly with the problems I faced. I also put my feet and hands to work. Throughout those long nights I circulated endlessly, going from room to room looking for problems. And I found them. Twice, once for each of the two least prepared nurses, I found IVs improperly set up and pumping air into a child's central lines. That, as I explain later, can be deadly.

Finally, I simply willed that nothing would go wrong that lay in my power to prevent. No matter how sleepy or exhausted I felt, I drove myself relentlessly. Nothing that was happening with these children would escape my attention. I would not relax for a single second.

Fortunately, the nursing administration soon noticed the incident reports filtering up. It ordered two of the three new nurses to undergo a second orientation. That and the fact that these nurses were learning from their mistakes eased my woes. Work returned to normal, and my stress level fell dramatically.

Months later, I received an unexpected benefit. For a reason I've long forgotten, one morning, rather than go to sleep as soon as I got home, I stayed up, planning to get the sleep I needed in the evening just before work. That was a bad idea. I must have turned off my alarm without waking, because the first thing I remember was the hospital calling. It was after midnight, and I was an hour late.

I lived nearby, so I dressed quickly and arrived about fifteen minutes later, expecting to be in big trouble. I wasn't. When I walked on to the unit, the shift supervisor was sternly warning the same nurses who'd gotten off to such a rocky start that they had handled the situation badly by not immediately calling her when I turned up missing. She directed no criticism at me, and to this day I wonder if anything about that oversleeping went into my file. I'd helped the nursing administration when it had been in a tight spot. It had returned the favor.

Next, we look at what could go bad on Hem-Onc, particularly with those complicated IVs.

6. Measure Twice

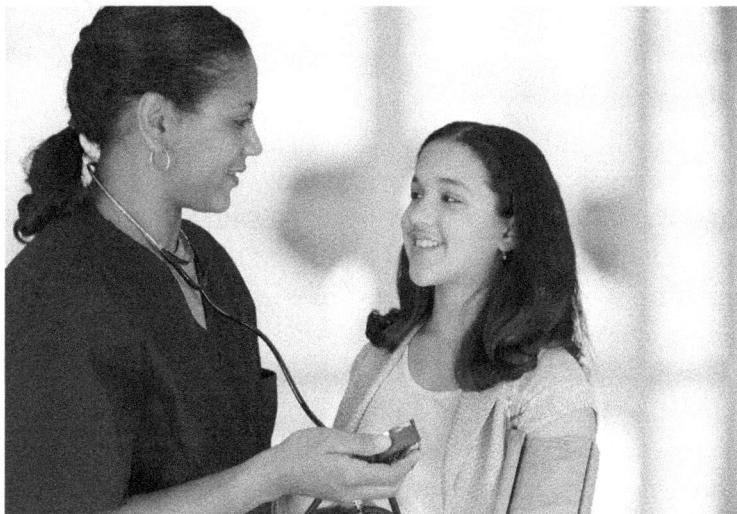

At this point, I should explain what typically went wrong, so you understand why it was so easy for those new nurses to make such serious mistakes. Our unit as a whole—Hem-Onc and the other two clusters—handled medical patients as opposed to those receiving surgery. That meant that roughly half our kids had an IV running. There was a practical reason for that. If a child could be treated with pills, he could probably be sent home. It was the IV that bound our kids to the hospital, even though they might not be that sick.

Almost all those IVs were simple, just a bag of normal saline (water with salt) running slowly. Typically, every four hours the nurse would run in a medication followed by a rinse to clear the medication from the line. That's easy, and there was little chance for error. Just get the medication and dosage right.

The IVs for kids with leukemia were far more complex. Even while I was undergoing orientation on days, I'd noticed the difference. Their IV poles typically had several bags hanging, along with two or even three IV pumps. When a child was first admitted, there'd be a large, golden yellow bag for chemotherapy or a smaller bag for the 'rescue' drug that followed a day later. Give them a poison, wait 24 hours, and then give the antidote was the essence of our chemotherapy. The toxicity of the chemotherapy also meant a bag with sodium bicarbonate to keep their urine slightly alkaline. In addition, there would often be a bag for running in medications such as antibiotics. We used a lot of antibiotics.

The complications did not end there. Since chemotherapy often left our kids feeling and eating poorly, there'd sometimes be a high dextrose (sugar water) bag to make up for the calories they were missing. It'd run only when no medications were going in.

Unfortunately, although high-dose sugar may keep hunger pangs away, we can't live on sweets alone. So kids on longer stays often had a large brownish-yellow bag with hyperalimentation fluids (vitamins, minerals, proteins, and the like), as well as a milky white glass bottle for lipids (fatty acids). Together, the two fluids—each with its own IV bag, pump, lines and sensor—provided almost all nutrients a child needed. Hyperalimentation (also know as Total Parenteral Nutrition or TPN) was a kindness. We didn't have to pressure these sick kids, who already had enough hassles, to eat when they didn't feel like it. But feeding them through their veins meant more complications for the nurse and more chances for mistakes.

Of course, no child would have all those IV treatments running at the same time, but almost every child had several. That meant a complicated maze of identical-appearing clear plastic lines running down from bags that looked almost identical, through several drip chambers, assorted IV pumps, and multiple sensors to the patient. Some fluids could be mixed, their lines passing though different pumps and joining at a Y-connector close to the patient. Some could not be mixed, so when one flow started, another had to be stopped. In addition, flow rates often needed to be changed. Adding to that complexity, different procedures meant different valves must be opened or closed. This was why many nurses felt they were caring for IV pumps rather than patients. They took care of the IVs, while I took care of the kids. It was almost true.

Those complications meant that a nurse whose only prior experience had been with a single IV line was way over her head coping with these numerous bags, drip chambers, pumps, lines and clip-on alarms. It was like someone who'd been trained to fly a single-engine light plane in the countryside suddenly being expected to land a multi-engine commercial jetliner through a crowded metropolitan airspace. Despite being sleepy, tired, and working in a dimly lit room, a nurse had to think through every move and recheck everything before leaving. The solution resembles the old adage carpenters have about "measure twice, cut once." The absence of training in always measuring twice, was one reason these new nurses made such serious mistakes. Before a nurse left a patient whose IV had been changed in any way, she needed to check every part of the IV system. With practice, that only took a few seconds.

That's where I came in. During those first three months, I'd watched and asked enough questions to learn those procedures. Life was more casual on night shift, so I was free to learn nurse-only tasks. I avoided giving medications, which I considered a no-no. But a nurse could go on break, depending on me to shift an IV that'd been giving a medication back to fluid maintenance at the right time.

More important, even before those unfortunate replacement nurses arrived, I backed up whatever my nurse was doing. When I came into a room, I'd take a moment to flip on the small flashlight that hung around my neck and trace the lines from bag to patient, making sure everything was as it should.

On Hem-Onc another factor dramatically increased the danger. Most of our IVs came with a serious additional complication—central lines. One of our doctors had invented a popular central line, and we were one of the first to use them with children getting cancer treatment. Installing a central line was typically the first step in their treatment.

You can see a central line in the picture of The Girl at the beginning of chapter 44. The line, made from rubber-like Silastic tubing, enters through the white patch on her chest. It runs just beneath her skin—notice the bulge—and joins with a large vein just before that vein returns to her heart. Where it enters the circulation is the key. Regular IVs connect into the peripheral circulation, smaller veins typically in the arm. A central line goes into major vein close to the heart.

For children with leukemia, central lines are absolutely wonderful. A child's veins are small and it's hard to keep them still enough for an ordinary IV to last more than a two or three days. That meant a terrifying poke every few days to start a new IV, as well as often-daily pokes to get blood samples. For kids enduring the horrors of chemotherapy, a central line that could stay in place for months meant an end to those pokes. For staff like me, who were already forced to inflict so much pain on helpless children, a central line was a wonderful blessing.

But central lines come with a serious risk. Air can be injected through them into large blood vessels that are only inches away the heart and brain. A bubble can then lodge in an artery, shutting off the blood supply to a part of the heart or brain. For our patients the chief risk lay with those dastardly IV pumps. If the wrong valve was open—an easy mistake to make in a darkened room— air rather than fluid would drawn in and pumped into a child's veins. That was the problem that worried me most when I worked with those ill-trained nurses. And because it was a relatively new problem for the hospital, we were still learning, slowly and laboriously, to cope with it. More on that later.

One incident was particularly disturbing. It happened after I caught air going into a child due to a mistake made by one of the two inexperienced nurses mentioned in the previous chapter. I instantly stopped the IV, moved the child into a protective position, and told the nurse.

Several weeks later I discovered that she hadn't reported the incident. Fear had led to secrecy and a cover up. Later, I'll write about the conflicts that arose when the mistake rate at the hospital reached disturbing levels. One reason was that recrimination had replaced mutual support. Mistakes led to anger, harsh criticism, conflicts, and fear, which led to still more mistakes. Rather than help others avoid mistakes, nurses felt under pressure to protect themselves by covering up their mistakes and finding fault with others. That was most unhealthy.

Incident reports like the one that nurse didn't file matter because they offer evidence of weaknesses in patient care that needs correcting. In our case, the weakness was a sensor clipped over an IV line to warn when air rather than fluid was passing through. For other types of patients, that was hard to get wrong. There was only one IV bag, one pump, and one line for that one sensor. But for the kids on Hem-Onc, that wasn't true. All those bags, drip chambers, pumps and lines made it easy to put that critical air sensor on the wrong line. The problem was so serious, as I was leaving the hospital was preparing at great expense to replace our IV pumps with a model less mistake-prone. It was also in the midst of a dreadful crisis I'll discuss later.

Next we look at what childhood leukemia is and what causes it.

7. LEUKEMIA EXPLAINED

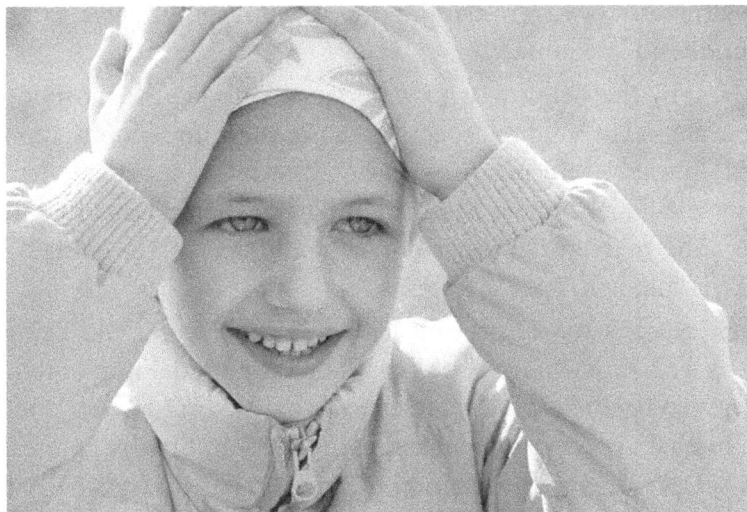

First, a disclaimer. I'm no expert on childhood leukemia and my experience with its treatment is now many years in the past. Today's treatments are more sophisticated, far better tailored to the individual child, and—most wonderful of all—often less brutal than those I experienced. That said, to understand what I will say, you must understand childhood leukemia and how it was treated when I worked Hem-Onc.

Leukemia literally means "white blood" because it involves rapidly multiplying, immature blood cells called "blasts," a shortened form of lymphoblasts. The name was chosen because, in the last stages of the untreated disease, those large numbers of rapidly multiplying white blood cells turn a patient's blood whitish. I've never seen whitish blood myself, but I have seen blood closer to slate gray than the dark wine red of normal venous blood.

Leukemia in adults can be a *chronic* disease, meaning the symptoms come and go, allowing someone to live for many years. Leukemia in children is almost always *acute*, meaning that without treatment it gets worse quickly, often killing within a few months.

At one time there was no effective treatment for childhood leukemia. Over a half-century ago, I was told, even physicians who suspected it would do everything possible to avoid that dread diagnosis. They'd exhaust every other possibility before doing a simple blood test to check for leukemia. Why? Because leukemia was a death sentence. No doctor wants to tell parents, "We can do nothing. Your child will die." Only in the late 1960s did a few specialists raise the possibility that, with the new treatments they were developing, it might be possible to actually cure childhood leukemia.

Judging by the children who were referred to us, the most common reason a physician might suspect leukemia is an infection that goes on week after week, refusing to go away. That's because those leukemic cells are selfish. They care about nothing but themselves. They rapidly fill the bone marrow, shutting down production of the normal white blood cells that help fight infections.

Other reasons for suspecting leukemia include a child being pale and tired with no obvious cause. That's because production of red blood cells has also been cut back. Another reason is pain in bones and joints caused by that excessive bone marrow production. Finally, bruising easily is a symptom, since production of the platelets that stop bleeding is also reduced. If you think of the bone marrow as a factory for blood, with leukemia it becomes a berserk factory turning out almost nothing but greedy, cancerous cells.

Of course, those signs may look like something else, and a misdiagnoses can delay treatment. Kayla, a gentle nine-year-old girl I cared for, endured weeks of joint pain that left her unable to stand. Her family physician diagnosed juvenile arthritis and tried to treat that. When his treatments failed, he referred her to an arthritis specialist at our hospital, who quickly sent her to us. What Kayla had looked nothing like arthritis. It was leukemia made worse by delay. She bore that terrible blunder with remarkable patience.

Before you blame family physicians and pediatricians for a missed diagnosis, keep mind that childhood cancers are thankfully rare. Leukemia is the most common form of cancer in children, but it's still unusual. In a typical year, only one or two children out of ten thousand get cancer. That's good news for children, but it does mean that the typical doctor isn't expecting to see cancer in his young patients. Often, it'll be one of the last things that comes to mind.

With childhood leukemia, once diagnosed, events move quickly. It wasn't unusual for a pediatrician to see a child in another state in the morning and make a tentative diagnosis that put that child and his parents on a flight to us that afternoon. Because the disease progresses quickly, our physicians wasted no time beginning treatment. When I came to work Sunday night, I might find a child finishing up chemotherapy who had not even been diagnosed when I'd left work Friday morning. Treatment moved that fast.

There was usually only one delay. When a newly diagnosed child arrived on Hem-Onc, there was a tense period as we waited for a more specific diagnosis. That's because there are three broad types of leukemia, depending on which immature blood cells have gone rogue.

The 'good' leukemia—if such a term even makes sense—was Acute Lymphocytic Leukemia or ALL. It's the most common type (roughly 60 per cent) and that's good because it was also the one whose treatment is the most successful. At the time I was caring for these children, the success rate was around 70%, odds many people with other cancers would be delighted to have. But those numbers still meant that about a third of our children would die. Since the sickest patients spend the most time in the hospital, the odds for children actually under our care were actually worse than those numbers suggests. On a typical night, I could assume that at least two of my young patients would eventually die. That I never let myself forget.

The second most common form of childhood leukemia is Acute Myelogenous Leukemia or AML. It's bad news and common enough (38 per cent) that there's reason enough to worry. Back then, I never heard success rates given, but my own sense was that at that time only about a third of those with AML were cured. It wasn't a happy diagnosis and was the one we hated to hear.

Beyond that, are a variety of other forms of leukemia that are either rare in general or rare in children. I took care of one such case, a girl diagnosed at six months with a leukemia so rare at that time the world's medical literature described only 32 cases, with hers being the youngest. She's Jackie, the little girl who is so special that she gets four chapters of her very own.

Once treatment begins, two words—both starting with "R"—become important. *Remission* is the good one. It means that there's no evidence from a child's blood or bone marrow that the cancer is still present. Doctors speak of remission rather than cure because no evidence doesn't necessarily mean no disease. The initial round of chemotherapy almost always puts a child into remission. It's how long that remission lasts that hints at the future course of the disease.

Obviously, the longer in remission, the better. Rather than keep patients in remission limbo forever, in the late 1960s, physicians chose to define five years in remission with merely maintenance chemotherapy as a cure. That allowed children and their families get on with their lives.

Unfortunately, there's nothing magic about five years. Near the end of my time at the hospital, I took care of a lovely sixteen-year-old girl who'd been in remission that long. Since the drugs that treat leukemia have terrible, long-term consequences, on this visit she was getting her last dose of maintenance chemotherapy. I encouraged her to move on with her life, but I now wonder if I should have kept quiet. Six weeks later she was back. Only suppressed by the maintenance chemotherapy, her leukemia had returned. When the leukemic cells reappear, it's called a *relapse*. That's the bad R word, the hated one.

In short, remission is good and eagerly to be sought, while a relapse is bad. A series of quickly occurring relapses can become a death spiral. A child doesn't have enough time to recover from the harsh results of one round of chemotherapy before needing another. At the time I was caring for these children, we had only one additional weapon in our arsenal, a costly bone marrow transplant. More on that later.

Now we'll look at the treatments available at that time.

8. No Magic Bullet

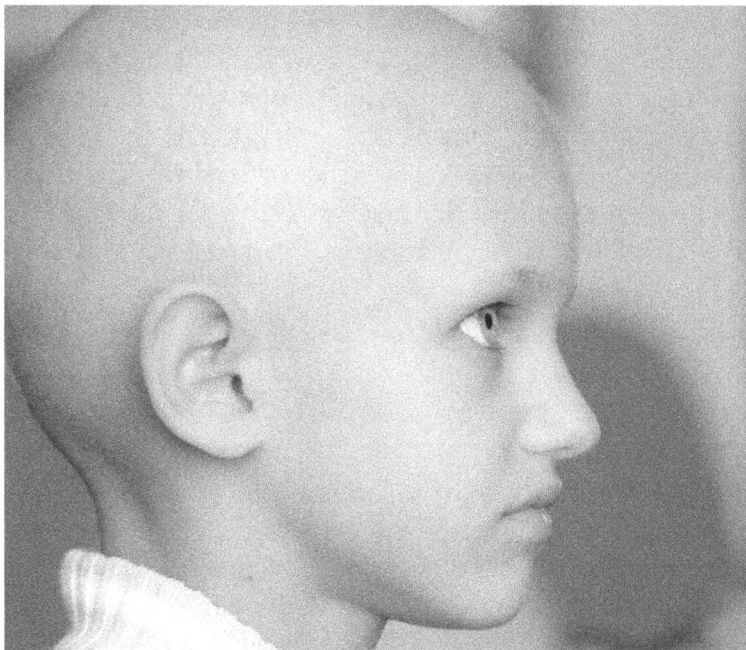

Normally, children with leukemia appeared to be only in moderately bad health when they came to us. They had symptoms that send parents to their family doctor with worried looks. Their child, they would tell the doctor, had a cold that wouldn't go away, mysterious bruises, or perhaps joint pain—little stuff with terrible implications.

It was our chemotherapy that transformed these children into the walking dead. Sadly, our 'magic bullet' wasn't very magic. It was more like dynamite. To destroy the rapidly multiplying leukemic cells, we used drugs that attacked every dividing cell, causing it to die and break apart. Our children's hair usually fell out and painful sores might develop in their mouths. Worst of all, their blood counts—red, white and platelet—would plummet to dangerously low levels.

Infections were a serious risk. In healthy people, a virus called CMV (Cytomegalovirus) is so wimpy, people often don't know that they're infected. In our patients, CMV could be fatal. In addition, the antibiotics we gave to fight bacterial infections could have unfortunate side effects. They destroy the healthy bacterial flora of a digestive system, which can lead to a fungal infection, mouth sores, and intestinal bleeding. Little in medicine is without bad side-effects, including antibiotics.

To be blunt, what we did to our young patients was awful. To save them, we had to risk killing them. That's why they looked so terrifying when I looked over at Hem-Onc during my orientation. At the time I was working with these children, doctors were trying to discover when a particular child could be treated less aggressively. The good news is that those efforts have borne fruit. Today's treatments are often less harsh and less likely to kill. But that wasn't true for the kids I describe here. We knew little, so we had to treat aggressively and thus harshly. To save them, we had to risk killing them.

The risks and the suffering involved in treatment meant that parents had to trust our doctors. I saw two cases where that trust was made even more difficult by the parents' background and beliefs. Their cases also illustrate how a child's past can make a big difference.

The first was a family living in a cabin deep in the woods of Washington's Olympic Peninsular. They had two delightful daughters, one about four and the other two. They were living what some would consider the most healthy life imaginable. They ate fresh fruits and vegetables grown in their parent's garden and had no television or video games to detract them from an abundance of sunshine and outdoor play. I still remember their robust health and the marvelous smell from a flat of garden herbs the mother brought on their first visit.

Despite all that natural goodness, however, the youngest of the two, whom I'll call Lily, developed leukemia, Fortunately, it was ALL, the so-called good one, but that still meant a brutal course of chemotherapy. Parents who would have never had let their Lily enter a room with cigarette smoke, now had to agree to let doctors flood her body with cancer-inducing chemicals. For a day we held our breath, wondering which they would choose.

They chose treatment, and Lilly's response taught me that good health is a marvelous gift. She breezed through chemotherapy better than any other child I cared for. Amazingly, she didn't even lose her lovely blonde hair. As far as I know, her treatment was successful. Her health certainly made a big difference.

The other patient was Bao, a boy about nine years old. His background was radically different. He had been diagnosed with leukemia at a Southeast Asian refugee camp and admitted to our hospital on a medical visa. Coming from a rural Asian background, his family's trip to America, to a large city, and to a state-of-the-art hospital must have been difficult. They had to trust foreign doctors who understood not a word of their language and knew little about their culture.

Complications soon developed. During the year I knew him, Bao rarely left the hospital for more than a few days. His health had been wrecked by persecution and starvation. Along the way, he'd acquired obscure tropical infections. I remember one morning when I was asked to stay over to transport him to a nearby university hospital to get radiation treatment for an infection in the bones of his jaw that had resisted all other treatment. "Radiation for an infection," I thought. "This is getting desperate." It was.

Shortly after that, I came into his room about 2 a.m. His infection was now so out of control, he was in a coma. In his mouth was a nasty fungal infection, a result of the heavy doses of antibiotics he was getting. He'd just had a bowel movement, so I decided to test his stool for blood, even though there were no orders for that. It was positive for the first time. That almost certainly meant the fungal infection had spread to his intestines, causing him to bleed internally. "This is it," I thought. "He's not going to make it."

A few days later as staff we were cautioned that no one quite knew how his family would respond when he died, but we were to be as understanding as possible. They took it quietly and resolutely. His death had been a long time coming. Given what he had been through, from the start his chances were far less than those for Lily.

All that suggests the obvious—that in an medical crisis a child's core health matters. Perhaps the best illustration comes from a seminar I attended at which a physician shocked his fellows by claiming to have found a cure for asthma. He went on to explain. Whenever possible, he had his patients, when they were in good health, exercise and build up their cardiovascular system. His goal was to get their heart and lungs working so well, that even after an asthma attack cut their breathing capacity by 50 percent, they'd still take in enough oxygen to not feel anxious or sick. Avoiding symptoms mimicked a cure.

Something similar was true for Lily and Bao. Lily was in such robust health that even when our treatment blew away perhaps 80 percent of her immune system, the remaining 20 percent could still fight off infections. On the other hand, Bao was desperately ill even before his leukemia struck. He'd been living in dreadful conditions on a poor diet for years and probably arrived in the U.S. already carrying the very infections that killed him. His chances were much worse.

For parents who're reading this book and worried that a child of theirs might get leukemia, that's the best hope I can offer. Those who treat leukemia are dedicated, caring, and capable people. The treatments they use are effective and continually being refined. As bad as it may seem, there are cancers far worse than leukemia.

But there is something you can do to prepare your child for leukemia or any other sickness. Encourage your child to eat, play and live as well as possible. That'll provide a reservoir of good health that could make a critical difference if some dread disease strikes. You don't have to live in a cabin deep in the woods to give them a healthy life, nor do you have to obsess over every little thing. Simply make a sustained effort to give them an active, healthy life. That will help.

9. Sharing Skills

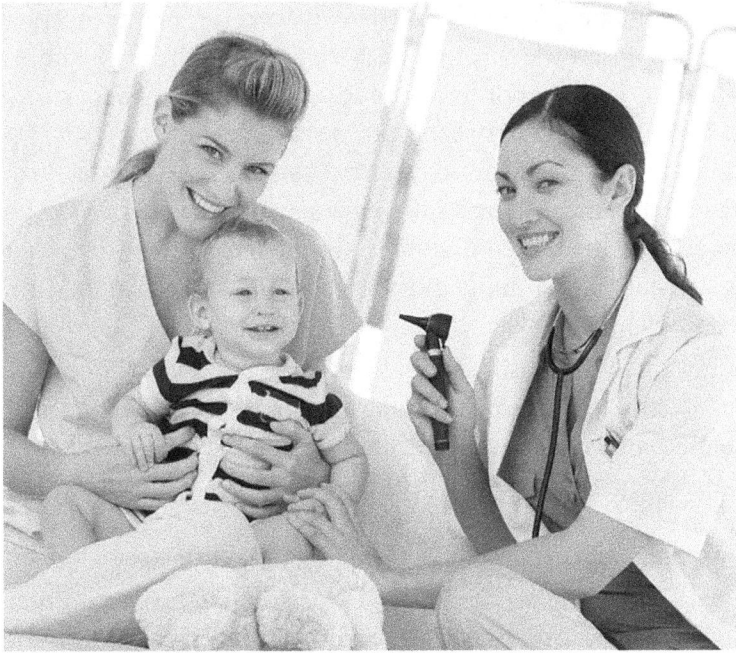

In the military, almost everyone is expected to learn the jobs of those around them. That makes sense. In combat, the person next to you may get killed or wounded, requiring you to take over for them in a instant. If you can't, events may go badly.

The death toll among hospital staff is much less, but the principle is the same. It helps to know more than your job requires. That's why it's great when those who work in hospitals want to expand their skills. What they see someone else doing, they want to learn. Sometimes that desire is accepted by co-workers. Sometimes egos intervene, and it isn't.

The result can be funny. While working at the hospital, I taught CPR to staff. The nurses—almost all women—didn't mind being taught by an aide or a guy. But one of my fellow CPR instructors told me of something hilarious that happened during one of his classes. When the lecture ended and the hands-on portion began, every male medical resident in the class quickly moved to his side of the room. He knew why. They didn't want his co-teacher, a nurse and a woman, telling them they were doing anything wrong. It was a sad but telling illustration of the male doctor versus female nurse silliness.

It was also pitiful. Such attitudes distort what ought to be a culture based on competence and mutual support. From top to bottom, those who work in a hospital need one another. I'll say more about that later.

I was fortunate. When I first began working at the hospital, the competency culture was strong. I was surprised at the skills the hospital was willing to teach me or to let me learn. The nursing department was willing to blur the line between nurses and aides, seeing both as part of a team. That was good. In today's terms, my EMT training, brief as it was, had qualified me to be a nursing assistant. The on-the-job training I received made me a skilled nursing technician without the bother and expense of school. I regularly did things that in some hospitals might be done exclusively by nurses.

For instance, the hospital taught me how to do peritoneal dialysis, often used with children with kidney failure because it's less gruesome than hemodialysis. In the latter, blood is removed through a vein, filtered, and then returned. For little kids, that's a terrible poke given two or three times a week through tiny veins. In peritoneal dialysis, a semi-permanent tube is inserted into the abdominal cavity, allowing its organ walls to substitute for a kidney. Special fluid is put into the abdomen, left there while it absorbs waste products from the blood, and then drained out. The process is repeated over and over, typically through the night. It takes longer, but isn't as invasive. No needles are involved, and kids can sleep through it.

Our hospital pioneered peritoneal dialysis for children, and those historical roots lingered on. I was told that there were peritoneal dialysis machines so well-designed that parents could use them in their homes with tap water. That may be why a large, four-bed room next to Hem-Onc that had been intended for dialysis wasn't being used at that time.

Families might have state-of-the-art equipment at home, but our own peritoneal dialysis machine was stone age. In fact, we joked that it was probably the world's first peritoneal dialysis machine. It was that primitive. A steel rack on wheels held large, five-gallon glass bottles on two levels, one high and one low. A complicated Rube Goldberg arrangement of timers and electrically operated valves opened to let fluid drain in and out of the child. Open high to let fluid drain into a tummy, wait about half an hour, then open low to let the fluid drain out. Repeat that through the night. On the sides of the bottles were crude, hand-drawn lines. My responsibility was to make sure those clanking timers and valves moved fluid in and out properly. When I did that, my nurse had one less thing to worry about. I enjoyed doing more, while she enjoyed doing less. A good arrangement.

Perhaps I should explain here what team care meant. When I worked at the hospital, most nursing care depended on it. With only rare exceptions, a nurse and I shared patients. She did certain things such as administer medications. I did others, particularly taking vital signs: temperature, pulse, respiration, and (when ordered) blood pressure. Only rarely did we break with that routine. Of course, that wasn't the practice everywhere. In other parts of the hospital, particularly the ICU, the totality of a patient's care was assigned to a single nurse.

Team care has advantages, the most important being that two heads focused on one patient are often better than one. Some problem with a child that I didn't catch might be caught by my nurse and vice-versa. It also meant that, while what we did was different, each of us could spot mistakes the other made. As I mentioned earlier, for nurses that usually meant making some blunder with those complicated IVs. That's why, when I entered a room, I flipped on my flashlight and checked IV lines. I got so skilled at that, it only took a few seconds.

In my case, mistakes often meant forgetting to do one of the myriad of small and constantly changing tasks my job required. The wee hours of Monday morning after a weekend off were particularly difficult. My eyes burned, my skin felt scratchy, and my head throbbed. All I wanted to do was curl up in an empty bed and go to sleep. I had to force myself to stay focused on the kids. Having a nurse around helped.

Working as a team also meant that we could cover one another's breaks on nights when there was time for one. Often, the only time my nurse could slip off was just after her 4 a.m. medications had gone in and their follow-up rinse (to clear out the last traces of the medication) had started. With charting totals due at 6 a.m. and meddlesome administrative staff arriving at the same time, that was her last chance to get free. Once I learned the routine, I could switch an IV from medication dispensing to fluid maintenance, giving her a half-hour head start.

That said, as an assistant I studiously avoided two things. The nurses knew that, if there was a medication mistake, they'd be blamed, so they didn't delegate that to me. Knowing that, I stayed away from dispensing them. Giving an IV med is easy. A child of eight could learn the procedure. What mattered were potential complications, especially of a wrong dose or an overdose. That required formal training I'd never had.

The other area I avoided were procedures that medicine calls invasive, meaning those involving inserting things into patients—catheters, NG (nasogastric or nose-to-stomach) tubes, edemas, and IV needles. All were skills I sometimes wish I'd learned, just in case I need to do them in an emergency. But it was also true that learning them wasn't best for our young patients. Why subject a child to something I would do badly the first few times, when a nurse who could do it much better was always there? Nurses must learn on someone because those tasks are part of their job. But those procedures weren't in my job description, so it was hard to justify upsetting kids with my newbie blunders. That's why I confined myself to pulling tubes and IVs rather than inserting them. That required less skill.

Later, I'll discuss how that training-centered, team-spirited, and co-operation-driven competency culture broke down and describe the disastrous consequences. For now, realize that at one time cooperation did exist and that it worked well.

Next, we'll look at pecking orders in a hospital. Yes, at certain times and places, the hospitals that many hold in such awe can bear a disturbingly resemblance to the cackling of a hen house.

My Nights with Leukemia

10. Pecking Orders

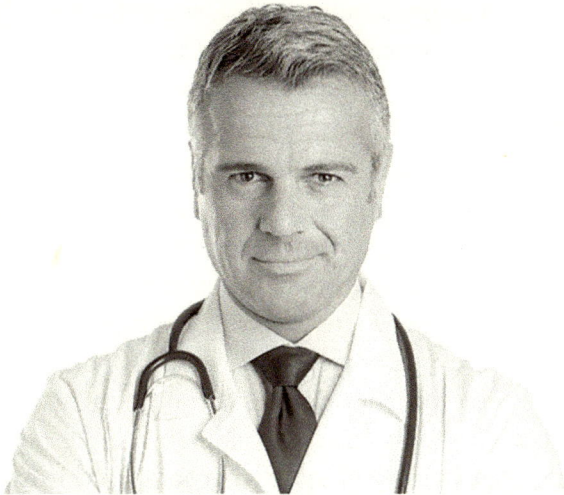

If there's a pecking order in a hospital—and there certainly is—then housekeepers are near the bottom, despite the fact that heir work is as vital as that of anyone else. A dirty hospital would be a deadly hospital. Most housekeepers I worked with didn't let their low status get them down. They had a job to do and did it well. One even proudly told me of an occasion when her lack of status made no difference.

She was busy cleaning outside the room of a child who was under strict isolation. Sometimes isolation is to keep infections away from a child with a compromised immune system. Our leukemia patients were in that situation. At other times it's to keep what that child has from spreading to other children. A rotavirus infection can spread like lightning through an entire hospital wing. Once we had so many cases that we ran out of isolation rooms and had to put kids with the same infection together. In either case, isolation must be taken seriously.

I forget which isolation applied to the situation this housekeeper described. What mattered was that two doctors had gone into a room that had signs clearly posted without observing any precautions. Thankfully not shy, she opened the door and called out to the two, telling them to leave immediately. One didn't take her remarks well, and began to say something along the lines of, "Who are you to tell us what to do." The other interrupted him, pointed out that they should follow the rules, and led the other out.

Later, that second physician took the time to thank the housekeeper. She'd reminded him of what had happened during his residency. He had been working in the emergency room when a young girl who obviously had an infection was admitted. Despite the fact that they knew they should take precautions, he and another resident worked over the girl as she coughed. Two days later, the young doctor he'd been working with died of what the girl had—a highly virulent bacterial meningitis.

Of course, there's no way to eliminate hospital pecking orders completely. It's born of an environment where some give orders and others follow them. But the pecking can be kept under control. The problem with status-driven, top-down orders is that they interfere with a healthy competence culture—one where everyone not only knows their job, but helps others to do their work well, much as that housekeeper did when she corrected those two physicians. At the heart of that is everyone treating fellow workers with respect. No one is God, not even a hospital's most senior physicians—despite what some may think.

At the time I worked there, the nurses were having much-needed success at getting doctors to treat them better, but the road was a rocky one. One area where new residents and new nurses clashed was in starting IVs, an area where both wanted to gain expertise.

Starting an IV on a small child is hard. Many won't stay still as they're being poked. That's why I often had to hold them. Their veins are small and soft-walled, so success requires a delicate touch. Despite that, many nurses were skilled enough to start an IV on their first try. That was rarely true of our neophyte residents. Some refused to delegate the job to a more capable nurse, arguing that they needed to learn. But pity the poor child whose parents weren't around to intervene.

One night I floated to Babyland, which is what we called the unit where the hospital put most babies up to their first birthday. There a resident—one whose stubbornness and lack of skill I'd already noticed on Hem-Onc—repeatedly tried to start an IV on a crying baby, before stalking off in disgust. Hands-on medicine differs from bookish medical school, and students who do well in the latter don't necessarily know how to handle the former. Failure often led the less emotionally mature residents to flee without a word to anyone.

I'd been the one who'd been forced to hold the baby through the ordeal. After he left, the baby's nurse came up to me and asked if he'd followed the 'three-poke rule.' The rule meant that if you couldn't start an IV in three tries, you passed the task on to someone more experienced. "Well," I grimly told her, "he tried in three places, but he poked a lot more than three times." That particular baby needed an IV, so she went into the room and came out a minute later, a big smile on her face. The IV was started, probably on her first try. The three-poke rule was an indication the hospital was changing. No longer was anything a doctor did right. Even he was only got three tries.

Another change lay in who was responsible for cleaning up a mess. Multiple IV attempts create clutter: abandoned needles, alcohol swabs, and paper wrappings. On one occasion, I was told, a couple of residents created a mess and then rushed off, one of them telling the other that cleaning up was "a nurse's job."

Unfortunately for him, that was now a no-no, at least for lowly residents. Good manners were invading an ancient autocracy. If a doctor really did have to answer an urgent call, he was expected to ask a nurse to handle his mess. According to the account I heard, it took only about an hour for word of that infraction to wind up the nursing chain of command, cross over to medicine, and then back down to that ill-fated resident, who returned to the unit and apologized.

Unfortunately, when I worked there, rules like those were still for little people. In the hospital's pecking order, residents were at the bottom of one hierarchy, often below the parallel rank of more experienced nurses. Senior physicians were at the top of that same hierarchy and not only didn't have to obey rules, some saw no reason to do so. The world they'd trained in had been clearly hierarchical and that's what it would remain until the day they retired. After all, what was a hospital going to do—fire them? They were the ones who brought in patients. So nurses gritted their teeth and consoled themselves that eventually new and better-mannered doctors would rise to the top. Maybe, maybe not. As the old adage goes: "Power corrupts. Absolute power corrupts absolutely." In a hospital, senior physicians have almost absolute power.

I saw a telling illustration of the Old School in a medical ethics class I later took. I knew our guest speaker from working at the hospital. He was one of the nation's top surgeons for children with severe disabilities. There was no doubt about his skills or his compassion for those children. But for him, nurses were different. How they felt didn't count. They existed to do as told.

Perhaps to shock us, he told us of a situation where a disabled child was in such severe pain, he ordered a massive dose of morphine. Thinking he intended to kill the child with what would normally be a lethal dose, the nurse refused to carry out his order. Ignoring her, he entered the child's room and administered the morphine himself. To us—but not to that nurse—he explained that he knew from experience that the child had a high tolerance to morphine and required that large dose. Upsetting the nurse hadn't bothered him in the least. In fact, he seemed to have enjoyed it.

That's Old School Medicine. Doctors give orders, while nurses obey. I not only disagreed with that, as you will see I believed that even aides like myself could dissent when it was clearly in a patient's best interest. As Thomas Jefferson pointed out, "a little rebellion now and then is a good thing."

Finally, the pecking orders in hospitals aren't just between different jobs. They also exist between more and less experienced staff. Almost all the experienced nurses I worked with were marvelous. They patiently answered every question I asked, however stupid. Many had amazing talents and had moved into specialty areas where they had the decision-making prerogatives of physicians. They liked that.

Unfortunately, there were other nurses who'd become older without becoming wiser. As you will discover, the worst clashes I saw at the hospital weren't between doctors and nurses or even between someone in a high position and someone in a lower one. They flared up between an older nurse who'd been stuck doing a particular job for many years and a new one who'd been doing it for a few months.

The results were dreadful. In the eyes of the old fogies nothing the newbies did was right. I came to suspect that some of these older nurses were unhappy with their lives and taking their anger out on younger, more enthusiastic, and often more talented nurses. They were driven by jealousy. I'll discuss that in more detail later. For now, just remember that nurses sometimes have problems getting along.

My Nights with Leukemia

11. ELI, THE FIRST TO DIE

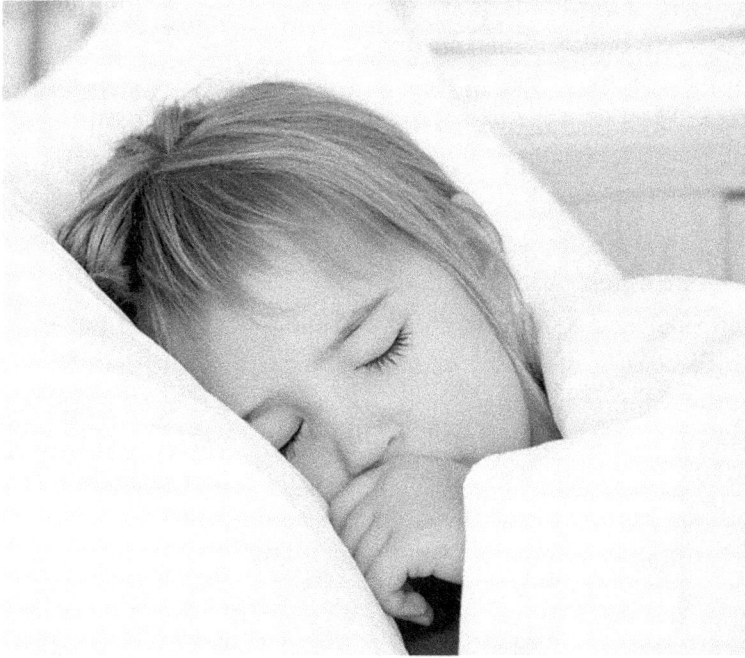

A long with getting good medical care, there's something else that matters to sick and frightened children. That's emotional support. Families matter throughout our lives, but they are absolutely critical for a child who's sick and in a hospital—particularly during those long and scary hours of the night.

While I was being oriented on day shift, I could see a boy dying of leukemia just yards away on Hem-Onc. The somber faces of the staff and the outsiders coming for one last visit told the sad tale. Still, that boy was fortunate. He was dying surrounded by an intact and loving family. Not all children face death that way. Some, I found to my shock, face dying alone or almost alone. That was the situation of the first child I cared for who died, a little boy I'll call Eli.

Eli was two years old. By the time he became my patient, all his chemotherapy options had been exhausted. We had no treatments left. In his own way, Eli understood that and was more terrified than any other child I cared for.

Each evening, I'd hurry though my start-of-shift routine with the other children to get to him. When I came into his room a little after midnight, I knew he'd still be awake. I'd pick him up, and we'd sit in a rocking chair. Every muscle in his body was so tense, holding him was like grasping a tightly coiled spring.

I would rock him back and forth, talking quietly. Slowly, his muscles would relax and his breathing would slow. After about half-an-hour, he would fall asleep. Then I'd rock him for another fifteen minutes to make sure he was deeply asleep before putting him in bed. Fortunately, small children can sleep soundly. If I was careful when I checked on him at four a.m., he'd sleep until morning.

I describe Eli as the first child I cared for who died but not as my first death because he didn't remain with us until the end. I never met his mother. She was single and apparently without family or close friends nearby. No one on staff held it against her for not staying with him overnight. His illness had been long and exhausting. She had a job with bills to pay and needed rest.

As Eric began dying, she took him home to be with her—probably against the advice of our doctors. That's when something happened that illustrates a point I can't stress enough. When a child is sick, single parenthood can be terrible and anyone who says otherwise is clueless or worse. Caring for a healthy child alone is hard enough. Caring for one who is dying is an incredibly difficult task. That was the situation Eli's unfortunate mother found herself in.

Later, I heard what happened from a friend who worked in the emergency room. As Eli slipped into a coma, his mother panicked and rushed him to our ER. She was so stricken, it took some time for the staff to quiet her down, discover who her son was, and learn what his situation was. To the extent that dying can be good, Eli's dying wasn't good. It came in a strange place surrounded by a distraught mother and confused strangers.

The situation was different for the first patient who actually died under my care. He was a boy of about three that I'll call Tommy. During his last days, both parents were able to stay with him.

With children, we didn't go for aggressive treatments with almost no chance of success. Adults can make a meaningful decision to go out fighting to the last trench, but children can't. It's usually cruel and pointless to impose one last and futile round of suffering on a child, particularly when the only motivation might be to relieve adult guilt.

But Tommy was an exception. Children with leukemia responded differently to the primary chemotherapy drug of that day, Methotrexate. He'd proved extremely tolerant to even high doses. Unfortunately, his leukemia was also tolerant of the drug, which was why he was dying. Our chemotherapy had done him little good, but his family decided to make one last, desperate attempt. As he lay dying, he would get a massive, round-the-clock dose of Methotrexate that wouldn't hurt and might help. Methotrexate works on cells as they divide, causing them to die. Maybe, if the treatment was aggressive enough, it would beat back his leukemia for a few months. For him, there was little harm in trying.

As a result, with his IV running fast, I was in and out of his room throughout the night, changing diapers stained yellow by the drug every half-hour or so. I did my best to enter quietly, but every time I came in, his eyes would open and look up at me. He wasn't tense like Eli had been. His parents were in the room and could comfort him far better than I. He illustrates the importance of two parents and an intact marriage. They were able to support one another and be with him until the end. Dying is never good, but dying can be better.

That brings up an important point. From time to time, I asked myself if, while caring for those children, I saw anything resembling the five stages of grief described by Elisabeth Kübler-Ross in her groundbreaking 1969 book, *On Death and Dying*. Her stages were: 1. denial, 2. anger, 3. bargaining, 4. depression and 5. acceptance.

I never did. Fear—or perhaps more like terror—I saw in the eyes of children such as Eli and Tommy. Being young, they knew little about death other than that it was something dreadful, like a monster stalking them in the night. That never changed or went through stages. Keep in mind though, that my focus was almost exclusively on the children. The middle of the night isn't a good time for talking with tired parents.

Others reacted differently, depending on their circumstances. In one girl, I saw something resembling bewilderment. She was a pretty girl of about eight with long, beautiful, light-brown hair. With all she had going for her, she had always been able to use charm to get what she wanted. Now she faced a cruel and unrelenting disease that not only paid no attention to her girlish charms, it made her lovely hair fall out. As a result, she seemed utterly lost. Worse still, she had AML, the bad leukemia, and her dying was sad almost beyond belief. Call that denial if you want, but it was worse than that. Defeat might be a better word. She died utterly defeated by her illness.

With other children, particularly the older ones, I saw something more like grim resignation than Kübler-Ross's final stage of acceptance. They were quiet, rarely speaking, and seemed at a loss as to how they should feel, so they said and did little. Today, so few children die of disease that our culture does little to teach them how to die or us how to accept their deaths. As a result, many die lost and silent.

Finally, some children were fighters who inspired respect from staff for their courage. Like the Welch poet Dylan Thomas writing to his dying father, they make clear that they will not "go gentle into that good night." Claiming that they were in denial or angry—sneering psychological terms—trivializes their determination to live or, in the case of one special little girl, to die on her own terms.

Pauline had severe cystic fibrosis, the same disease that killed one of my cousins, and she was dying from it at four. With an antibiotic-resistant infection raging out of control in her lungs, our doctors gave her only two days to live. We didn't treat cystic fibrosis on Hem-Onc, but an exception was made for her because we knew how to care for dying children.

Five days later and seeming to be in a coma, she was still with us. Her parents wisely decided she could sense where she was and was refusing to die in a hospital. They insisted on taking her home and were proved right. Ten minutes after little Pauline reached home, she let herself go "into that good night." Call that what you will, it doesn't fit into neat psychological stages. For issues of life and death, good literature is often better than the social sciences.

By far the most impressive illustration of refusing to die was the Jackie I've mentioned before, first diagnosed with a rare form of leukemia at just six months. Her desire to live was so great, it shaped her treatment. Within a few days of being admitted, she was in the ICU, battling so many problems the doctors only gave her a small chance of ever leaving our hospital alive. Yet there was no talk of ending her treatment. As one ICU nurse told me, her struggle to live was so obvious, no one thought of giving up. That's not denial. That's courage and determination even in someone very young. She was a most brave little baby.

Those I worked with made similar observations about dying children. The nurse whose responsibility was to deal with the social needs of these children and their parents came closest to the truth. She spent far more time talking with families than I did. When I asked her if she'd seen any of Kübler-Ross's five stages, she told me that she didn't think either these kids or their parents had time to go through stages. Events moved much too fast for that.

She was right. With childhood leukemia, diagnosis moved quickly to treatment and with treatment came hope or at least the illusion of hope. If treatment then failed, events again moved quickly to an end that left little time for stages. That's why doctors prefix the name for the childhood leukemias with "acute." It moves fast—terribly fast—often too fast for either a child or parents to adjust.

Next, I'll describe the larger societal background to issues that resulted in a little boy like Eli being left all alone, dependent on me to rock him to sleep.

12. Alone in a Storm

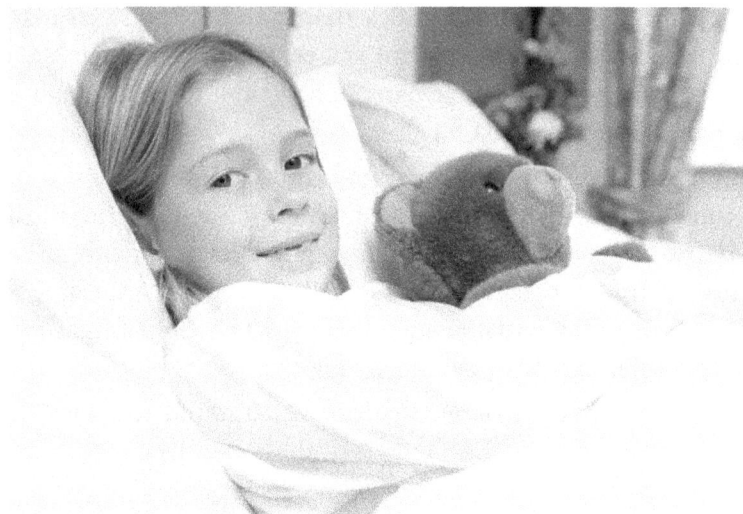

Perhaps NOAA should have fired whoever wrote the weather report about the winds on the lake being 10 to 15 knots that afternoon. After all, NOAA's Pacific Northwest regional headquarters was less than a half mile from the ramp where I launched my sailboat. You'd think it could get its own local weather right.

Their report lured me away from writing and got me to hitch my sailboat to the truck and head for the lake. The predicted wind speed, I thought, would be perfect for sailing—not too fast or slow. But the mistake was also mine. Before sailing away from the dock, I should have noticed windsurfers off a nearby beach. The wind was blowing so furiously, most were unable to stay up for more than a few seconds.

By the time I was 100 yards offshore, I knew I was in big trouble. With most of the 22-mile length of the lake to build up speed, the south wind was actually 20 knots gusting to 30. In physics, twice the speed means four times as much force exerted on my sails. Spray from the bow blew back almost horizontally to where I was seated in the stern, stinging my face. That near gale force wind was far more than my little San Juan 21-foot sailboat could handle without double-reefing the mainsail. But it was too late for that, in fact too late for almost anything I might do but desperately try to stay in control.

The only good news was that a little over a mile to the south lay the longest floating bridge in the world. Its giant pontoons, continuous except for two small openings for boats to pass through, were taking a terrific beating. But for that, the lake would have been battering my little boat with four-foot waves. Unlike a sailor on the open sea, I only had to contend with that dreadful wind. That was enough.

Unable to see any alternative, I headed across the lake to a small cove on the eastern side. Sailboats go fastest on a beam reach, which is broadside to the wind. With a thirty-knot wind on my starboard beam and my boat heeled far over, I've never sailed faster. My little boat may have looked pretty to those crossing the battered bridge in the storm, but it didn't feel that way to me.

The cove on the far side wasn't an answer. It was filled with anchored boats to dodge and the hill to the south only partially block the wind. One moment I'd be in complete control. The next, a gust would hit and I'd be headed for an expensive yacht, my boat heeled over so far water was pouring over the sides into the cockpit. Compounding my woes, I broke the extension attached to the tiller that had allow me enough free movement to reach through the hatchway into the cabin while steering. Now I couldn't leave the tiller for even a second. I was nailed to the stern of my boat.

At the heart of my troubles lay an unfortunate fact. Virtually all my problems would have disappeared if there'd been two on board. One could manage the tiller, while the other reefed the mainsail, prepared an anchor, or jumped, rope in hand, onto the dock of a waterfront home. Surely, I told myself, no one would begrudge me tying up at their dock for few hours in this awful wind.

After about thirty minutes, I grew tired of playing Dodge the Yacht and headed back out onto the lake. At least there I faced more predictable horrors. Unfortunately, the wind wasn't showing any sign of letting up. I needed to get ashore before I got exhausted or made a mistake that hurled me overboard. With almost no other boats on the lake, I'd be in serious trouble in the water. Sure, within a few minutes someone would notice my out-of-control boat and call the Coast Guard. But rescuers would take time to arrive and would have no way of knowing where I was in all those chilly waves.

My options were few. The easiest escape was to run before the wind. In a storm, sailing with the wind at your back *feels* much better. Rather than smash into waves, each one comes rolling up slowly from behind. But that comes with a heavy price In about an hour, I'd face the lee (downwind) shore at the lake's north end.

There my hopes were few. In the northwest corner of the lake was a small sandy beach on which I could land. But that raised that one-of-me problem again. How could I steer my boat and get into the boat's cabin to crank up the 400-pound, lead-filled keel that extended four feet down and kept my boat stable? Raise it too soon, and the boat might roll over. Leave it down, and I'd run aground as I approached the beach.

An alternative was a small river that entered the lake's northeast corner. Once up it, I'd be partially sheltered from the wind. Ah, but again there was a hitch. The channel to the river was well marked, but it was several hundred yards long and only about fifty feet wide. Stray out of it and I'd run aground in that high wind. I'd done my best to rig my boat for single-handed sailing, but sailing that way in a storm was a disaster.

The only other option was to return to the launching ramp I'd left. But how could I dock when the dock itself was exposed to this wind? The usual technique is to sail toward a point downwind of the dock and, just before reaching it, turn into the wind and feather (release to swing free) the sails, halting the boat as it comes alongside the dock. Then I could jump onto the dock with a line in hand and tie the boat off. In moderate winds that's easy.

But this wasn't a moderate wind. I made a few trials and judging when to turn into the wind proved impossible. The moment I turned, the boat came to a halt, making my rudder worthless. Pushed back, the boat was hard to control. Again, I was stymied because the captain and crew were only me. A second person could have leapt onto the dock with a rope while the boat was moving.

I took a little comfort from another time I'd been on the lake. With skilled supervision, I'd done the right thing. I was in a 26-foot ocean-going yawl built for rough seas and crew to a seasoned captain. A similar storm was raging and what he told me to do made my blood run cold. He wanted me to steer his prized boat into the teeth of that roaring south wind and guide it though the smallest of the two passages under the floating bridge.

Why was I worried? Because sailboats can't sail directly into the wind. Instead they must tack on either side of the wind, sailing no closer than about 45 degrees to the wind's direction. I could see the opening from where we were and tell that we couldn't make it through it on our current port tack (sailing southwest). He told me not to worry, that he'd tell me when to throw the helm over and take up a starboard tack (sailing southeast). So we entered the dark passage under the bridge with the wind howling, the boat heeled over, and headed directly for a huge concrete piling. As we got closer to that piling, there was still no word from him. Finally, when it was only a few yards ahead, he told me to turn, which I eagerly did. With the momentum of the boat carrying us forward, we came around on the new tack just as we broke out from under the bridge. I could breathe again.

Later, he told me why he'd waited so long to turn. The wind blowing under the bridge was unpredictable. If we'd turned earlier, we might have gotten caught in an eddy and his boat could have stalled, leaving us without forward movement and no way to steer. In that storm, his boat could have been smashed to pieces in seconds. As terrifying as delaying that turn felt, waiting until the last second was safer. The moment we turned, we were clear of the bridge and in clear air.

Unfortunately, no experienced captain was with me that other day, and even someone ignorant about sailing could have offered two willing hands. After considering my options and finding them all grim, I finally hit on a solution. Two teen boys were out on the lake enjoying their family's ski boat. Employing a persuasion technique just shy of "You don't want me to drown do you?," I got them to tow me into wind, allowing me to drop my sails. Then they towed me alongside the dock, where—not having to control my sailboat—I could jump ashore, rope in hand. That worked, and I waved a most grateful thanks.

My experience that day without a crew or experienced captain is a chilling parallel to what it's like to be the only involved parent of a child battling a serious illness. But there is a critical difference. The stress I had to bear for a couple of hours is stress they have to bear for months on end. That should bother you. I know it does me.

Keep in mind that why that problem exists. Life is not like math. Two people aren't twice one. Often, two are ten times as capable as one. One can be overwhelmed with what two could manage with ease.

For the parents of a sick child, it matters less *how* they divide the load than that they *can* divide it. One pair may share everything, cutting the work of each in half. One parent, typically the mother, may take on almost all the burden of caring for the sick child, while the other manages the rest of their life, including the other children and working to support them. That was the most common approach. Finally, a child's parents may switch roles every few weeks. I saw all three while I worked on Hem-Onc. What was done is not as critical as that two were doing something that'd be excruciatingly difficult for one. Extended families are even better, with grandparents giving parents a much needed break.

Other family circumstances work far less well. I saw cases where there was a single parent, almost always the mother (as in Eric's case) who was struggling, often heroically, to cope with her child's illness while managing the other areas of her life, including earning a living.

Even more disturbing, there were cases where there was *no* parent or relative offering a child love or support. Not a single one. During my 26 months at that hospital, I cared for three children who were dying with little or no family involved. No child should die like that—not ever.

As those tragedies unfolded, I made no effort to assign blame. A child's illness often came too late to fix broken relationships. In most cases, I knew little or nothing about a child's family history nor did I go searching for who was at fault.

Look at what is happening in our society, and you'll understand why. A parent can end up single for any number of reasons, including death, divorce, and never marrying. Others may have alcoholism or drug addictions that render them incapable of being a good parent.

I didn't apportion blame because I didn't believe those choices—even when foolish or selfish in themselves—were made so a sick child would suffer. I have trouble seeing a mother get divorced simply to deprive her daughter of a father during a serious illness. Parents get divorced for other reasons, and then an illness happens. Bad, but not an intentional bad. Nor does a father say, "two years from now my son is going to get diagnosed with leukemia, so I'll evade my responsibilities then by becoming a hard-core drug addict now." That's not what happens.

To understand what does happen, look at the numbers. In our society, millions of people have broken or never formed families and troubled lives that leave them and their children vulnerable in a major crisis. Even in the best of times, many barely get by. That's bad and something we must correct. But only a small proportion of those—statistically only one out of thousands during a particular year—will find themselves in the situations I describe here. It's unfair to lay the blame on one person for a terrible situation when there are thousands of others who're living much the same lives, but don't happen to have a child with leukemia.

Remember my sailing adventure. I went out on the lake to enjoy 10 to 15 knot winds, and instead got hit with 30-knot gusts. I had made a mistake, a stupid mistake, and I was paying for it. Something like that was happening with these families. A mistake had left those families less able to cope with disasters. As a result, they were being overwhelmed by a situation they didn't anticipate and certainly didn't want.

As a society, we need to deal with the many reasons why we have so many families with but one parent or even with no properly functioning parent. That's rough in even the best of times. It becomes incredibly difficult when there is a child involved struggling with a serious illness. But it does no good to burden still further families that hit by rare events such as childhood leukemia. We need to fight the broader societal causes, rather than the occasional consequences. Our society needs to change, so every family is better prepared for a seriously ill child or other crisis.

I'll talk more about fractured families later. Next, we look at the wonderful little boy who loved trains.

13. Bobby, The Train Boy

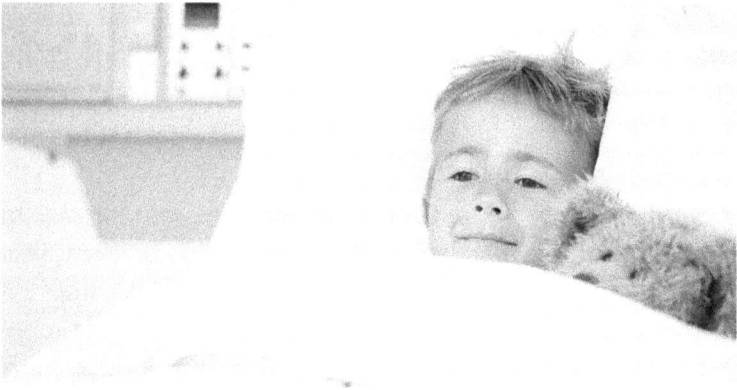

At the time, what happened made no sense. It was a little after midnight and the resident assigned to Hem-Onc was wrapping up her work, no doubt hoping to slip in a few hours of sleep in her brutal 32-hour shift. "Do you think," she asked me, "we should run another C&S on Bobby?"

Bobby was the 'Train Boy.' About four years old, but mature beyond his years, his nickname came from a cassette recorder on which he would play, over and over again, the mournful sounds of distant train whistles. Perhaps, like Johnny Cash's song, "Stuck in Folsom Prison," it expressed his wish to be out in the world having adventures rather than always lying sick in bed. The song opens with these lines:

I hear the train a comin'
It's rollin' 'round the bend
And I ain't seen the sunshine
Since, I don't know when.

But that freedom was not to be. Even before Bobby was born, his bone marrow had not produced red blood cells. His mother's blood kept him alive in the womb. Since then, he'd depended on regular transfusions. That wasn't good, so he needed a bone marrow transplant. That meant us, since at that time we were one of the few hospitals doing them on children. With him, there'd be no need for the usual lethal, whole-body dose of radiation to kill off his own blood cells. The procedure itself would be simple. The difficulties came later.

The transplant itself went well. But immediately afterward, an infection appeared. At first, it didn't seem that bad, merely spikes in his temperature. His doctors put him on antibiotics and ordered the first C&S test. As I mentioned earlier, the C was for *culture*, to see if a lab could grow a bacterial culture of his infection. The S was for *sensitivity*, to see which antibiotic killed that infection.

I thought of telling that resident, who was both pretty and intelligent, "Don't ask me. Orders for tests are your responsibility." But she was serious, so I decided to help. I checked on the hospital's computers. The C&S from two days earlier, when Bobby's infection first appeared, had come back negative a few hours before. That wasn't unusual. Sometimes a blood draw didn't catch germs on the prowl. I told her another C&S made sense, after which she wrote out the order.

Only later did I realize that what she'd done made more sense than I'd thought. Given that the unit was all-nurse on days, she probably thought she was asking an experienced nurse rather than an aide with scarcely any formal training. After all, our uniforms looked the same. You had to look closely at our name tags to spot the difference.

Unfortunately, this doesn't end happily. When I came to work the following evening, Bobby was gone. His infection had turned serious, so he'd been transferred to the ICU. The following day he died just before the results of that second C&S—the very test I had recommended— came back. This time, the C&S had tagged the antibiotic he should get. Unfortunately, it wasn't one he was getting. With nothing to go on, his doctors had ordered two broad-spectrum antibiotics. His infection fell between the two. A few hours too late, they discovered their mistake.

For a long time, I pondered Bobby's death. Working night shift, I rarely saw, much less had anything to do with decisions. They were made while I slept by physicians I barely knew, giving them an other-worldly quality. Someone decided what to do, and we did it. The results, for good or ill, followed fatalistically. That created an attitude that doing a good job meant carrying out their orders to the letter rather than playing a role in those decisions.

But in Bobby's case, I'd been part of a decision that had life or death consequences. Would that resident have followed my lead if I'd suggested not running a second C&S? Almost certainly not. The need was obvious, particularly since the first test had come back negative. She was merely asking me to support what she'd already decided. Yet there were the two of us, in the wee hours of the night, making a choice that—had it gone just a little differently—might have saved the life of that wonderful train-loving boy.

That experience helped me grasp the difficulties our Hem-Onc doctors faced when, a few months later, I went to hear an epidemiologist give a breakfast talk on antibiotics. Several childhood cancer specialists—the distant bosses I never formally met—were there. You could tell how powerful they were by the fact that two were breaking the hospital's firm no smoking rule so flagrantly, one nurse loudly moved as far from their smoke as possible. And no, I can't explain why a cancer physician would chain smoke. Perhaps it's the "think they are God" syndrome. Some doctors believe the rules don't apply to them.

I did agree with their heated response to the young epidemiologist though. Like many specialists, that expert saw prescribing the right antibiotic as a complicated affair. The cancer doctors had no patience with that. If they discovered that an immunocompromised child had a serious infection at 8 a.m., they wanted to be able to write out an order for effective antibiotics five minutes later. Bacterial cultures have their place, but cultures take too long. Better to shoot from the hip than to do nothing. Anything that improved their aim was welcome.

Of course, that wasn't the whole story. Any process, no matter how long established, can be improved. The more I thought about what happened to little Bobby, the more I wondered why happenstance played such a large role. Why was that resident making a decision which was so important? Why did an order for a C&S result in a single blood draw and a single, often-fallible test? Why didn't it result in a series of orders repeated each shift until a positive result came back?

After all, wasn't finding the cause of the infection what we were after? We weren't testing to see if little Bobby had an infection. We knew that, and one failure did not change that. We desperately needed to know what was causing his infection. If that took several tests, then several tests it should be.

Yes, tests cost money. But perhaps a hundred thousand dollars had already been spent keeping little Bobby alive. Now that we were so close to a cure, what difference would a few hundred more dollars make?

Remember, people aren't numbers. Cost-benefit analysis, so beloved by some in the darker, more bureaucratic corners of medicine, fails to take into account factors that matter more. Unfortunately, in any money-centered analysis of Bobby's situation, his death comes cheaply. It was keeping him alive that was and always would be expensive.

Nothing came of my thinking. Perhaps at some level in the hospital those topics were discussed, but I wasn't privy to how I could inject myself into that. I'm sure the hospital's lead physicians were aware of my existence and of my nursing student co-worker. Capable staffing was one of their concerns. But feedback from us wasn't a part of medical care as they saw it.

To the extent that I could imagine a solution, I remember thinking that it should be computer-driven. Computers are like the little wind-up pocket alarm I used to remind myself to take follow-up temperatures. They're great for mindless repetition. One C&S order, entered into the hospital's computer system, could trigger a series of nursing orders, perhaps one each shift, until a successful lab result triggers cancellation and perhaps a 'this is the right antibiotic' message to the physician in charge or the resident on duty.

That's easy to do today. Unfortunately that wasn't easy with the technology we had then. Our medical care was paper-driven. Doctor's orders were written on standardized sheets of paper with carbon copies sent through a pneumatic tube system. Our state of the art wasn't that versatile. The computer system we used was little more than a bulletin board. True, data from lab results were automatically dumped from lab equipment into the computer, as one lab tech proudly explained to me. That meant I could look the results up from anywhere in the hospital, as I did with Bobby. But nothing more complicated than that could be done with a system that primitive.

Today, the situation is far brighter. I've never been someone who believes computers can replace people in every area. Machines are good for doing things we do badly, including remembering to order a series of tests. Our minds are better at other things. Given sufficient experience and good sense, we have an uncanny ability to see more than the evidence seems to indicate—to unconsciously pick up on a dozen seemingly insignificant events and conclude that something serious is happening. We call that intuition, and it's not something a computer does well.

I had yet to learn about intuition. My first glimmerings of its importance came with Binky, the amazing little boy that God made.

14. The Boy that God Made

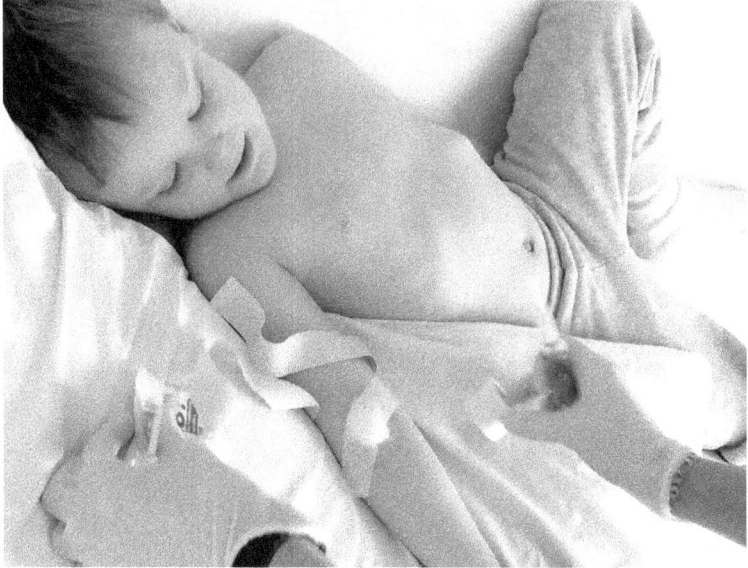

The first time I went up to Binky's bed, I saw a handmade sign someone had placed at the foot. It read, "I know I'm somebody, because
God don't make no junk." At the time I didn't know the words were
from the black gospel singer Ethel Waters, born as the result of the rape
of her young mother. I just knew that someone—perhaps his mother or
his nurses—considered this little boy special. They were right.

Binky had Prune Belly Syndrome. Those who have it—almost all are
boys—have few or no abdominal muscles, resulting in a tummy that
can look as wrinkled as a dried prune. In Binky's case, his tummy was
enlarged and his legs and arms were thin, making him look like the
Kermit the Frog toy he often had in his bed. While I knew him, he was
so weak he had to be propped up by pillows. But I've seen pictures of
him from home at a time when he was strong enough to stand.

Numerous abdominal complications come with the syndrome. In
Binky's case a diaper had to be placed close to his belly button, because
that's where his urine dribbled out, one drop at a time. He didn't have a
bladder, and I was also told he had only one kidney.

Kids with disabilities this severe often grow up quickly because they
face problems that would overwhelm most adults and spend a lot of time
with adult caregivers. That was certainly true of Binky. Few adults could

have managed the great courtesy and kindness he displayed to staff. I remember one situation as if it were yesterday.

With so much wrong inside, keeping Binky properly fed was hard. At times he needed a NG (nasogastric) tube running from his nose into his stomach so something like baby formula could be given. That was no big deal in itself. Those who treat it as something extraordinary and call for it to be discontinued in patients they don't want to live for other reasons are talking nonsense. The tube is as ordinary as a spoon or a baby bottle and is used for much the same purpose.

Since Binky had caught up nutritionally, an order had come to pull his NG tube. The tube is soft and flexible, so it doesn't hurt when in place. But there is a gaging sensation as the tip is pulled up through the throat, so I was trying to do that as quickly and gently as possible. Amazingly, frail little Binky—despite all he was suffering—displayed more concern about my feeling bad about the process than he did for his own comfort. Like I said, he was a most special boy.

As his health waned and waxed, Binky was in and out of our hospital. One visit would have a major impact on how I thought about my role. About a third of those who have Prune Belly Syndrome die of kidney failure, and that's what began happening with Binky. His single kidney was failing, so an effort was made to find a diet that would put as little stress on it as possible. One night I noticed—although not as well as I should—that he was breathing very fast, gasping about fifty times a minute rather than the usual dozen or so. The importance of that didn't register in my mind. I merely charted it like I'd been taught to do. I was still learning that I needed to do more than my job description required.

When I came to work the next night, Binky had been transferred to the ICU. As a nutritionist would later tell me, while trying find a diet that did not stress his kidney, they'd forgotten to include enough protein. Without protein, his frail body had begun to consume itself. That rapid breathing I'd recorded had been metabolic acidosis.

Binky spent a miserable six weeks recovering in the bright lights and beeping monitors of the ICU. I mentally kicked myself for not being more aware and assertive. Yes, sending out an alarm *that* night would have made little difference. But I still should have noticed and spoken up. On other occasions, quick reporting might matter more.

After that, it was several months before I saw Binky again. Then one night, as the evening nurse was giving report, an alarm went off and a

Code Blue light began flashing outside a room just a few yards away. Binky, I discovered, was in that room and had just stopped breathing. The evening aide had triggered the alarm so the code team could come, restore his breathing, and keep him alive long enough for his family to reach the hospital. Technically, he became my patient a few minutes later, but that aide, bless her sweet heart, stayed by his side, holding his hand until his parents arrived. Much is said about the inappropriateness of treatments that bring people back from the brink, but we should never forget that those same treatments can also allow someone to live long enough to die surrounded by those who love them. That's good.

Events soon demonstrated just how true that sign at the foot of Binky's bed had been. He was about four when he died and hadn't lived long enough to make many friends in the wider world, so his family held a small, private funeral. But they also knew that there were many at the hospital who'd grown to respect and love him, so they arranged for a memorial service for us led by the family's pastor.

When I first heard about the service, I wondered who would attend. His family understood our shifts well, so they picked the best possible time, which was early afternoon. But that only meant that attending was equally difficult for all three shifts. Those working days needed to find someone to come in early. Those working evenings needed a day nurse to stay over until they could get to work. For people on nights such as me, attending meant waking up at a time our bodies would regard as 3 a.m.

After the service, when a group of us went from the chapel to his grave site, one nurse asked me if I'd counted how many nursing staff were there. I hadn't, so she replied, "Twenty-four." With other kids, the most staff I'd seen attend a funeral was six. Despite his short life, Binky had become most special to those who knew him. We came to say that his life mattered, and it did. He really was the boy that God made.

Binky's kindness to us illustrates something that took me many years to understand. Why did some children, despite all their pain and suffering, show so much thoughtfulness to those around them? They didn't have to do that. Everyone would have understood if they'd been grumpy or even exploded in anger. Time after time, these children would thank me for doing some little thing, and I'd have to restrain myself from saying, "Oh, that's nothing. They pay me to do this." Only after much thought did I realize what I had been seeing—something very special.

Imagine for a moment that you're a child with an illness that will soon take your life. You're not wealthy, so you can't think of all the charities your accumulated millions will fund. You're not successful, with a long life of accomplishments behind you, nor are you famous, with millions of adoring fans eagerly awaiting news about you. You're only a little kid who has just begun life and yet you're dying. All you will accomplish in the rest of your life will take place over the next few weeks in a small circle around your bed and with the few who enter that circle.

That's what I was seeing with those remarkable children. They were giving meaning to their short lives by being kind to us. We were all they had, and by allowing them to be kind to us, their lives mattered.

For those who'd like to know more about Binky and the wonderful example he offers, I've included his chapter in *Hospital Gowns and Other Embarrassments* as the very last chapter of this book. That chapter and the book as whole offer excellent advice for anyone who is hospitalized and wants to take control of their hospital stay. You might want to read it.

Finally, those of us who've been given far longer lives should never forget the greater gifts and opportunities we've received. We've been blessed with much more time in which to do good. We should use it well. As Jesus said, "Whom much is given, much is expected."

Next we'll look at the debates surrounding medical care given to severely disabled children such as Bobby and Binky.

15. Special Children

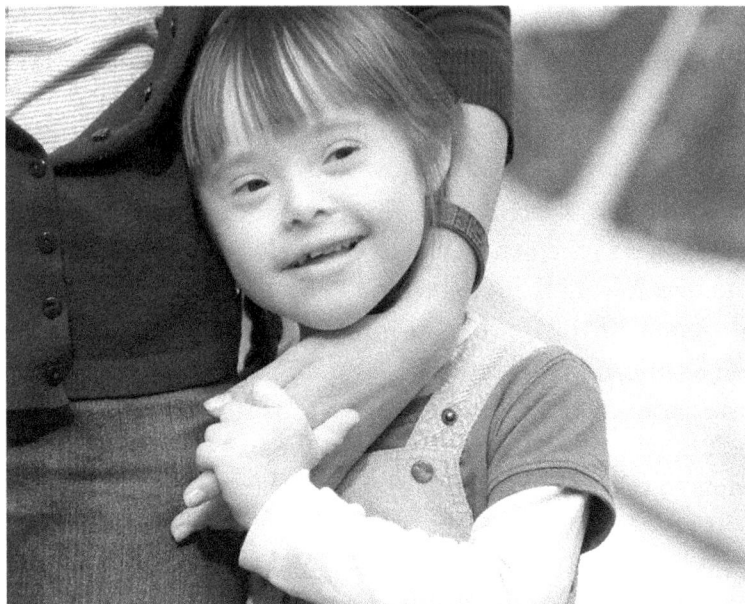

Today, some question the money that's spent on patients such as Bobby, the boy who loved trains, and Binky, the boy that God made. "We knew from birth that they would live short and difficult lives," they claim, "so why waste money on people like them? Look at the poor quality of their lives." That same utilitarian calculus also lies behind the denial of heart and other hollow-organ surgeries to children born with Down syndrome like the little girl in the photo above.

Their reasoning assumes that what these people value most—social status, professional credentials, and large incomes—are the measure of all things. When these bean counters are experts from prestigious universities or powerful government agencies, terms such as life expectancy, quality of life, and costs to society constantly crop up. In words Oscar Wilde once used to describe a cynic, these are people who know "the price of everything and the value of nothing." They forget that the worth of a human life isn't measured by a professional resume.

I have little patience with such people. "Fine," I'm tempted to say, playing the devil's advocate. "If we're getting rid of people who have difficult lives, let's start with the rich and famous who're unhappy. They're not only miserable themselves, news stories about their chronic woes—

their latest romantic breakup or divorce—make their fans unhappy too. Why not spread cheer all around by giving them a quick and painless death? It'll end their misery and all the pain they cause. Then we can pat ourselves on the back for our great kindness. We might even sell their property and give their wealth to charitable causes. What could be wrong with that?" By the utilitarian calculus I just described, nothing.

My tongue-in-cheek advocacy doesn't end there. "And if we need to limit rising medical costs," I'd continue, "why not direct our attention to aged politicians and senior government officials who've retired? The financial advantages of ushering them into the Great Beyond are substantial. With children born less than perfect, the only costs society bears are a few years of medical care, much of that covered by voluntary donations to children's hospitals. We aren't funding luxurious homes, expensive cars, or costly vacations—just a hospital bed and a few nurses.

On the other hand, if those high up in government died a few years earlier—although still after long lives—that'd help solve our budgetary woes. We'd save substantially on their medical care costs and, even more important, the much greater cost of keeping them in a comfortable re-tirement. We wouldn't even need to change medical practice much. We could just "No Code" these VIPs, perhaps refusing to treat any illness more serious than sniffles—although using the appropriate drugs to make their accelerated deaths as painless as possible. We wouldn't want to be unkind, after all. That'd save us more than enough money to care for wonderful kids such as Bobby and Binky.

Of course, those arguments will get you nowhere. These people are masters of hypocrisy and the double-standard. Their quality of life ar-guments are only for those like Bobby and Binkie. It's expensive, state-of-the-art care for them, but little to no care for the little people, partic-ularly when those little people are actually little.

Other revealing thoughts flood my mind. In grade school I remem-ber being impressed that the U.S. Army physician Walter Reed (1851–1902) researched the spread of yellow fever and developed a vaccine for it by exposing himself to the disease. Today, I'm not impressed by those who want to use others for experiments in medical cost containment. "Try the ideas on yourself first," I want to shout. Start with experts in academia and government bureaucracies, along with members of Con-gress and their senior staff. Establish a maximum cost for their care and cut off anything beyond that. Only last of all, after everyone else has been drawn into that grim, cost-containment web, should we turn to children with disabilities, children who—unlike those experts—bear no responsibility of the larger issues.

That is, if matters go that far. The advantage of cost curtailment from the top down is that, if it proves a bad idea, it's not likely to spread far or last long. Start at the bottom, and you can be certain that it will expand upward as far as the depravity of our political process permits. It won't be limited by any concerns for kindness or decency.

I can give a telling example from my own experience in academia. Leaping a bit into my future, after I left the hospital, I began graduate work in medical ethics at the University of Washington's medical school. "Studying law in the medical school," I jokingly called it, since my primary professor had a J.D. (*Jurius Doctor* or doctorate in law).

To enrich that experience, I took a course in law from the philosophy department, taking care to audit it, so I could say what I wanted. The professor proved a champion of the ideas I've described above, resulting in some interesting personal conversations.

Concerning children with Down syndrome, he told me "we have enough of those." I can only assume he had in mind a quota, official or unofficial, on how many such kids should be allowed to enjoy life—and enjoy life they do. Those I've known with Down are almost invariably happy and sociable. The Dr. John Down, who first describe the syndrome in 1866, referred to their "congenital inability to hate." Surely, our society could use more people like that.

Ah, but this professor did not agree. As we stood outside his office one morning, I decided to test him from a different angle. "Suppose," I asked him, "there's someone with severe, impossible-to-treat manic-depression. For 364 days out of the year he's utterly miserable, cruel to those around him and regularly attempting suicide. Then one day each year he enters his manic state and creates a single great work of art. Would you want to get rid of him too?," I asked. "No," he said quite firmly. "Revealing," I thought to myself.

At the time, I wasn't quite sure what lay behind his seeming illogic. That coffee-sipping, politically active, *New York Times*-devouring philosophy professor seemed to have little of the real philosopher in him. Some ethical systems talk about maximizing happiness, which could be used to justify getting rid of unhappy people. But I have trouble imagining an ethical system that would deliberately get rid of happy people, while forcing those who are unhappy and want to die to live on in utter misery just for an occasional painting. That seems hideously cruel.

The closest I can come to making sense of what that professor and his many kin believe is to imagine them preparing, ever so diligently, for a visit by a superior civilization of space aliens. In the presence of such creatures, a young man with Down syndrome who can do little more than clean cafe tables might prove an embarrassment, while that briefly brilliant artist would not.

And yes, I realize that they're not really thinking about visitors from space nor are they literally trying to keep up with intergalactic aliens. What they're actually doing is judging our society from what they think is a higher platform and drawing conclusions similar what a race of technologically advanced space aliens might adopt.

To grasp their beliefs, this may help. Ask yourself what the opposite point of view is to that disgruntled professor and his quota-setting fellow-believers? I think it was best expressed by a friend who had a child with disabilities so severe, her little girl would never be anything more than a baby, able to feel simple happiness and sadness. "Someday in heaven," the girl's mother told me, "my daughter and I will talk about our lives, and she will say, 'Mother do you remember when this happened. And we'll both laugh." Eternity provides an answer to issues that are never resolved in this lifetime. That's why those who lack eternities—such as that professor—get into such a dreadful mess. Every problem must be corrected in the here-and-now even if that correction involves killing on a massive scale. That attitude is one reason why the twentieth century was so horrible.

Starkly stated, those are our choices. Either we strive to evolve in order to impress some three-headed, blue-skinned, tentacle-waving race from outer space, should they ever decide to visit our obscure little planet. Or we can imagine a future life in heaven, where all our imperfections are corrected, even those of children such as Binky and Bobby.

We've looked at two special little boys. Next we look at a little girl who was also special, although she came into my life about six months after I left the hospital.

16. ANGIE, THE HI GIRL

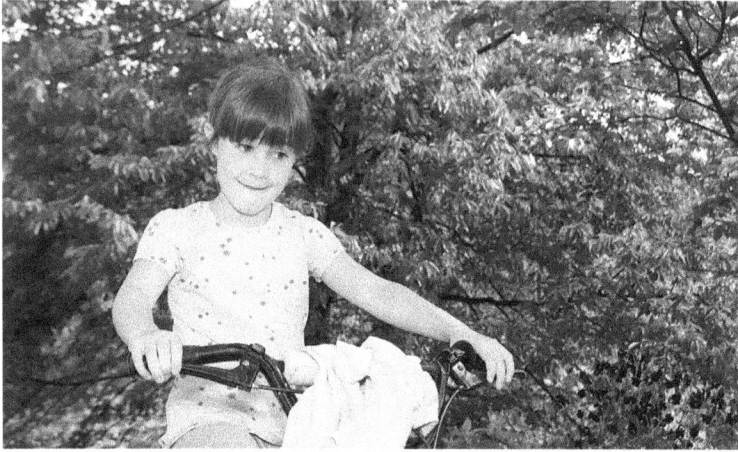

All of us decide based on our experiences. For that philosophy professor, his definitive experience was a fleeting encounter with friends who were the parents of a boy with Down syndrome. That was the source of his nasty remark about having of "enough of those." That's because it's hard to hate those we've never met. Bigotry requires at least fleeting contact with those hated. Anti-Japanese-American sentiment during World War II, for instance, was closely linked to already existing hostility toward immigrants from Japan on the West Coast, where most had settled. At the same time, those who hate often take care to make sure their experiences of the Hated Other are shallow and fleeting. That explains segregation and quotas.

Fortunately, my experiences haven't been shallow. In fact, I've known kids with far greater problems than those with Down syndrome. While studying medical ethics, I volunteered at a child development center on campus. The staff assigned me to a classroom with children who, I was told, had severe behavior disorders. "Oh my," I thought to myself, "in the social sciences they water down terms, favoring vague and inoffensive words. What must these kids be like to have severe behavior disorders?" I imagined padded cells and straitjackets.

Most, it turned out, had autism. The six boys, all around eight years old, had that diagnosis, and all were severe cases. None spoke, and only one seemed to understand what I said to him. One of the two girls was Rita, the little four-year-old who had been kept locked in a closet by a crazy grandmother. She didn't know how to talk, but I could sense that inside her was a little personality eager to break out. Unlike those boys, she wanted to join our world. When I welcomed her as she came off her little yellow bus, she would sputter and want to be hugged.

My life-changing experience came on the first day when the class's other girl, a cute, energetic, dark-haired little six-year-old, who looked much like the one pictured at the start of this chapter, came up to me and said, "Hi." Staff watching from behind a one-way mirror later told me that her eyes had locked on me the moment I'd entered the classroom. Angie wanted me for her friend, and that's what we became.

The squishy, social sciences term for Angie was that she was 'developmentally delayed.' That wasn't quite right. In her motor skills, she was, if anything, ahead of her age. She had no trouble darting about on a bike around a crowded playground. Socially, she was much like other girls her age. It's an age when many girls dote on their daddies. In fact, that's what she first called me—"Daddy." "No," I told her, "I'm not your daddy." That's when I first began to understand her. Tell her something was not so, and she learned quickly. I never had to say that again.

Angie's difficulty lay in learning broad new concepts. She'd been assigned to a severe behavior disorders class, staff told me, because when she first arrived, she had been wild and uncontrollable. Then some wonderful person taught her a single magic word, "Hi," and she quickly became angelic. She'd been wild, it turned out, merely to get attention. With that word, she could get attention of a funny sort. Staff called her the 'Hi girl' because initially her side of a conversation was little more than saying "Hi" over and over again. When she said that, people gave her attention. That's what she craved more than anything else. Although in the same class with those autistic boys, she was their exact opposite.

Learning to say "Hi" proved to be the key to teaching her something that seems obvious to us but that she'd not grasped before—that the sounds people had been making around her for years had meanings. Recall the moment when a blind and deaf Helen Keller first connected the water running over one hand with her teacher writing "water" onto the palm of her other hand. Angie was much the same.

Once she grasped the significance of sounds, she began to learn words as quickly as other young children. After I'd been there for a few months, we collected all the words she'd said and found the total was rapidly approaching a hundred. At about a hundred words, a speech expert told us, she'd begin to form simple sentences. That proved true. Shortly afterward, Angie pointed to a man walking his bike across a lawn and said to me, "See the man and the bike."

Angie's problem wasn't with learning itself. She could learn words as easily as most small children. It lay with grasping the new and abstract, such as that the sounds people make are a way to communicate.

That was true in other areas too. One day I watched a tester grow increasing frustrated trying to discover Angie's IQ using a standardized test. "You won't get far," I felt like telling her, "because Angie doesn't understand that you want her to answer questions. She wants you to tell her what to say, then she will say it." Angie understood teaching. We taught her all the time. But testing was different. It was a new game, one she didn't yet understand.

Angie had the same difficulty with personal names. When she called me "daddy," I resolved to teach her my name. That shouldn't be hard, I thought. After all, she had learned "bike," so she should be able to learn "Mike" easily. To make the lesson into a game, I'd take her hand, point it at her, and say, "Who is this?... Angie!" Then I'd point at myself and say, "Who is this?... Mike!"

It didn't work. Week after week, I repeated our little game several times a day when we were together. She'd smile, but seemed to regard what I was doing as yet another mysterious adult activity. Finally, I realized that she was held up by her 'learning something new' problem. Understanding the purpose of words had been the key to her learning to speak. But what she'd learned was that words describe *kinds* of things like bikes. That's why she'd called me "daddy." Daddy was her word for men she liked. What she hadn't learned was that some words only apply to one person. That was a new idea, one she'd not yet grasped, so I kept up my little game.

Then one day, after about six months, she began to play the game herself. "Who is this?," she said, pointing at me. When I said "Mike," she began calling me by my name. I made sure she understood that was a Big Thing by picking her up, whirling her around, and praising her.

When I came in the next day, the staff told me that she'd learned the names of six other people. She'd finally grasped an idea that'd be a great help to her in the future—that people had names unique to them. It was then that I realized I'd created a problem. Pointing and saying, "Who is this?," isn't the proper way to ask someone's name. But teaching her the right way to ask for names was trivial. The hard part had been getting across that each of us has a special name. Between her first "Hi" and her later "Mike," she'd learned almost all she needed to know about relating to people. The rest was details.

Angie should help you understand the mindset of that quota-setting professor. Taking six years to learn your first word or six months to discover that people have personal names isn't likely to impress visitors from an advanced galactic civilization—at least not one that values efficiency, progress, and technological expertise above all else.

Quotas for children with Down syndrome and similar problems make sense to such people because having more than a few of them around as tokens isn't seen as efficient. Taking months to teach a child your name does nothing to progress the human race toward its ultimate destiny in an artistically gifted and technically sophisticated utopian state. For an illustration of how such people think, read Aldous Huxley's *Brave New World,* where people are placed into categories, with strict quotas on how many in each are born in state-run baby hatcheries. Huxley, it seems, knew people much like that philosophy professor.

George Orwell described that futuristic, obsessed-with-planning mindset to near perfection in *My Country Right or Left* when he wrote of the science fiction writer H. G. Wells:

> If one looks through nearly any book he has written in the last forty years, one finds the same idea constantly recurring: the supposed antithesis between the man of science who is working toward a planned World State and the reactionary who is trying to restore a disorderly past. In novels, utopias, essays, films pamphlets, the antithesis crops up, always more or less the same. On the one side, science, order, progress, internationalism, aeroplanes, steel, concrete, hygiene: on the other side war, nationalism, religion, monarchy, peasants, Greek professors, poets, horses. History as he sees it is a series of victories of the scientific man over the romantic man.

For the exact opposite of H. G. Wells, think of J. R. R. Tolkien and his old-fashioned little hobbits. Perhaps that is why those with a Wellsian bent hate Tolkien, who was a language professor and poet.

We turn now to a different patient, a fascinating little boy who was an exaggeration of many boys his age.

17. Josh the Wild

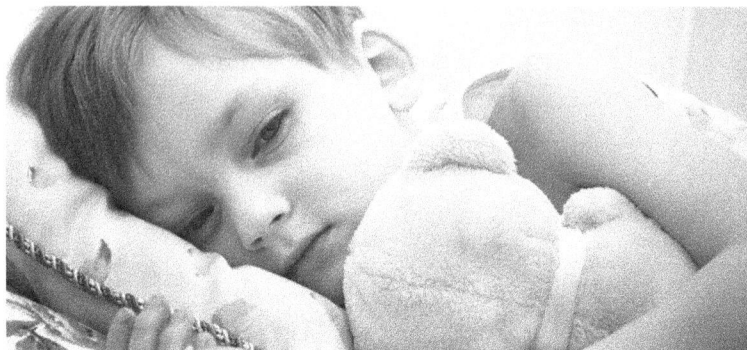

Sick kids are not all alike. Some are marvelously well-behaved. Others are far from sweetness and light. I first I heard about this boy when the evening nurse described him as the "wild man of Borneo," referring to someone in a freak show at an old-time circus.

Josh was about two and hated being confined so much, she said, he'd already tried to climb out of his crib several times. That's no small feat. Hospital cribs have slick metal rails and tall sides. One restraint vest, normally more than enough for a small child, hadn't been strong enough for this sturdy boy. He'd ripped out the cords that held him down. Now he had two restraint vests, and they were barely enough.

When I first checked on him, he lived up to his reputation for rebellion. His diaper hadn't been changed quickly enough, so he'd taken it off and was smearing poop on the rails of his crib. "He's going to be interesting," I thought. That proved an understatement.

Josh's illness has slipped my mind—perhaps a blood disorder such as aplastic anemia. Over the next few months, he was in and out of our hospital. Each time, he trusted us a bit more and became a little less wild, although remaining as stubborn and determined as ever.

One visit was especially memorable, because it helped me realize just how unflappable I'd become. It was about three a.m., and a rare moment with nothing to do had descended on our unit. I was talking with two nurses at a nursing station when the call light outside Josh's room went on. Since a light usually meant aide work, I responded.

Normally, I didn't turn on the florescent lights when I entered a room. The light from the hallway was enough to find my way about and, if I needed more, I had a flashlight. Bright light made it harder for a child and his parents to get back to sleep. But in this case, as soon as I entered the room I sensed something was wrong and flipped on the lights. What I saw was shocking. Every square foot of open space was covered with small, bloody footprints. They were all over. I called for my nurse and took a quick look at Josh, who was seated on the hideaway bed next to his mother. He was alert, aware, and perhaps even a bit too delighted by the fuss he'd created. "Good, he's not in shock," was my instant diagnosis. No need to hit the code button. Like I said, I'd become unflappable.

Talking with his mother, we soon understood what'd happened. For a reason that now escapes me, Josh was on a fluid restriction, meaning that neither we nor his mother were to give him anything to drink. The only fluids he got came in a carefully measured dose through his IV. He got thirsty, and, Josh being Josh, he decided to do something.

He'd been sleeping with his mother, so he got up without waking her, intending to get himself a drink from the sink. That's when a detail matters. His IV wasn't the usual needle in his arm. Like many of our long-term patients, he had a soft, flexible central line that went into a large vein on his upper chest.

As Josh went for the sink, he didn't bother to take his IV stand along, so the connection between it and his central line popped open. Fortunately, blood comes out slowly when that connection is severed, so it simply dribbled onto the floor, a drop at a time. Judging by his many bloody footsteps, he must have wandered around the room for at least ten minutes, trying to discover some way to reach that appealing water tap. Finally, with both socks soggy with blood, he realized something was wrong. He awoke his mother and handed her a blood-soaked sock. That's when she hit the call light, and I entered the story.

In the end, there was comic relief for all involved, including his briefly terrified mother. To make sure all was right, we called in the resident, the same lovely one who'd asked me about running a C&S on Bobby. She concluded Josh was fine. Even a small quantity of bright-red blood spread out looks shocking, but he hadn't lost enough to do any harm. We did take one precaution though. He was already scheduled to receive red blood cells later in the day, so I persuaded her to let us run the blood in during the night just to be safe. Maybe, I thought, that will help a bit with his thirst too. Josh always made caring for him an adventure. I sometimes wonder what happened to him.

Josh's real-life story, involving a loss of blood, is a good place to comment on a film I once saw that, judging by an Internet search, is the original source for a host of urban myths. It's one of the most moving film shorts I've seen. Based on the clothing worn, particularly the physician's double-buttoned white uniform, it dates from the 1930s and, based on the quality of the film, probably from the late 1930s.

As the film opens, we see a little girl of about four who is lying unconscious in a hospital bed. She's pale and breathing weakly, so it's obvious she's in deep shock. A distinguished physician is standing beside her. He turns to her brother, who's about six. The boy is lying in the next bed, alert and watching his little sister. He's healthy and well.

Your sister will die, the doctor, tells the little boy, unless a someone who's closely related donates blood for her. No blood banks yet exist, so he tells the boy that he's their only source of blood, and the only one who can save her life. The boy agrees to give his blood, so the doctor sets up an apparatus to transfer blood directly from him to his sister. After a few minutes, the transfusion is complete, and we see the little girl began to wake up. She's going to recover and live.

At that point the physician turns to the boy, who seems to be struggling to say something. Encouraged, the boy asks the question that's been on his mind since he agreed to give blood, "How long," he wants to know, "before I die."

Of course as adults we know better. We know that the amount of blood the doctor took wasn't enough to kill the boy. But we should never forget that our ways of looking at the world often aren't those of little children. Some small children really do believe that, like they have only so many fingers and toes, they have only so much blood. What was taken for lab tests and the like, they think, could never be replaced. That can be terrifying, and is why that boy believed giving blood to his sister meant sacrificing his own life.

There's a lesson there. We should never forget that the fears of small children aren't our fears, nor is their courage like our courage. Something that's of no importance to us may matter greatly to them.

Next, we'll look my struggle to do my work well despite being surrounded by so much dying.

18. A Place for Dying

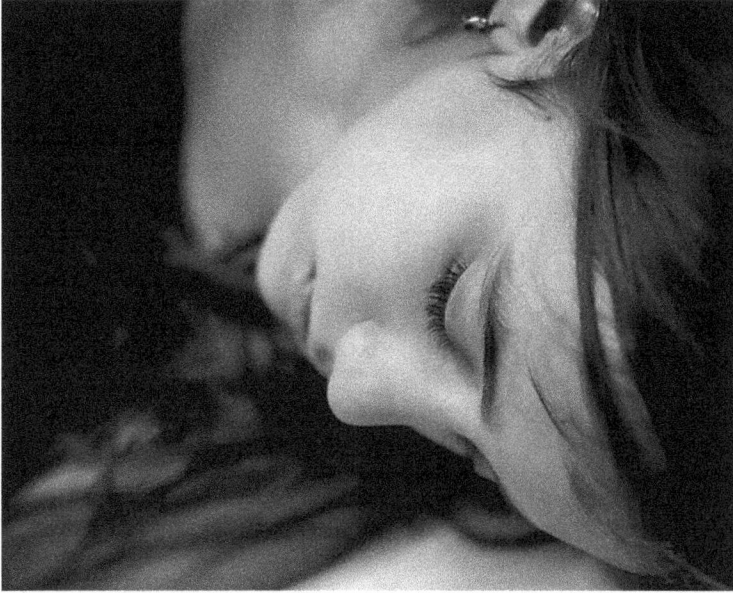

In addition to taking care of children with cancer, Hem-Onc was the place where the hospital often sent children who were dying for other reasons. That lent a tragic 'death row' air to the place. Any night I might come to work and discover that I had a dying child among my patients.

Sending such children to us made sense. Situated in the hospital's far southwestern corner, we were as isolated as any wing of a major city hospital could be. Our staff could cope with dying children, or they wouldn't be there. In addition, the parents of children with leukemia were facing their own issues of life and death, so another dying child didn't create trouble. Finally, because of the severity of the illnesses and the immunocompromised situation many of our children were in, few visitors dropped by. That left us as isolated as if we were behind locked doors. That led to special situations.

One night, I arrived and discovered that we had a patient with a rare genetic syndrome called *Cri du chat*, French for "cry of a cat," because children with it have a unique way of crying that's like a cat. Its cause, a missing portion of the Chromosome 5, was discovered in 1963 by Jérôme Lejeune, the gifted French geneticist. It's slightly more common in girls, but this was a boy of about four.

According to the chart, this boy, whom I'll call Charlie, had a mental age of about eight months. I never observed that or heard his unusual cry. Behaving like his mental age would suggest, he'd choked on a toy, been rushed to the emergency room, and was now dying with an erratic breathing pattern called Cheyne-Stokes, which is a characteristic of people with severe brain damage.

Since there was nothing my nurse could do for him, he became exclusively my patient. At home, he had been cared for by foster parents who probably had several other foster children, so no family member would be with him during his last hours. I was to be his last friend.

There was little I could do other than drop in as often as possible, talk softly to him, and make sure he seemed relaxed and comfortable. Then, to illustrate how dense I can be, about 3 a.m. I went in and noticed that he had thrown up on his sheepskin pad. As I began to clean the mess, I realized that he wasn't breathing. Given how loud and unusual his breathing had been, I can't explain why that wasn't the first thing I noticed. I went to tell the nurse he was dead.

What followed illustrates how responsibilities differ in a hospital. My reasoning was simple. He wasn't breathing, therefore he was dead. That's true as far as it goes. When the nurse arrived, she went a bit further and held a stethoscope to his chest for about ten seconds, confirming his heart wasn't beating. That's another indication of death. Then she left to call the resident on duty. He came down and—as I watched—made a much more elaborate confirmation of little Charlie's death, listening at various points on the boy's chest for about a minute with his expensive stethoscope. "He's the one who must sign the official death certificate," I told myself. "He must get this right."

On another night, there was a mysterious new admission, a boy that I remember as having greatly advanced leukemia, although it retrospect it might have been aplastic anemia. I mentioned him earlier as the eight-year-old Ralph with a dangerously low platelet count.

Ralph seemed mysterious because children dying of cancers and other blood disorders were almost always children we knew well. In our region, we were the hospital where such kids were treated. And yet, although he had obviously been ill for a long time, no one seemed to know anything about him. As far as I could tell, he had never been a patient of ours. If he lived nearby, why hadn't we treated him? If he was being treated by another hospital, why wasn't he there?

In this case, Ralph wasn't coming to us to die. Only his father was with him and, if his family had known his end was near, others might have been there. We intended to coast him through the night, although with a platelet count of 6,000 (normal is around 300,000), he had no ability to clot his blood. The slightest rupture in the tinniest blood vessel could bring out-of-control bleeding.

I was told to keep him as calm as possible. That's why a mild pain in his foot triggered an immediate order for IV morphine. That brings yet another mystery. If getting upset was bad, I asked myself that night, why didn't we sedate him? And since platelets were waiting for him in the pharmacy, why didn't we give them that night? Why wait? His nurse and I could give them as easily as day shift. In retrospect, the whole affair was filled with unanswered questions.

By that point, I was familiar enough with what a low platelet count meant to know that entering into his room was like carrying a blazing torch into a warehouse filled with explosives. I needed to check up on him, and yet what if my presence triggered the very upset that we were trying to avoid? It felt like walking on egg shells. Whatever I did might be wrong. Not visit, and something might happen that needed to be discovered. Visit and I might trigger something disastrous.

In the end, we received a sad lesson in dying badly. A century ago one of the founders of Johns Hopkins Hospital, William Osler, called pneumonia the "old man's friend." He meant that, of all the ways someone could die, pneumonia was one of the most gentle. Unlike a heart attack or many cancers, it wasn't painful in itself because morphine blocks any discomfort caused by a lack of oxygen.

That's why, although I've written a book about J. R. R. Tolkien's simple-living little hobbits, I'm less a critic of modern technology and its powers than some of his fans. There's no reason to be nostalgic about our past. We don't have to be slaves to our technology. The ability to *do more* carries with it the ability to *do the right thing* in more situations. In Osler's day, there was little that medicine could do to make dying less painful for many illnesses. Pneumonia really was a friend because morphine masks respiratory discomfort well. Today, we have many more such friends. That means that, while we often can't prevent death, we can at least ease the dying.

For childhood leukemia, the dying has not always been good. Decades ago, childhood leukemia often meant a terrible death. Unable to keep a child's blood counts up with transfusions in an era before well-organized blood banks, they often died precisely as Ralph died that night in front of his father—horribly and terribly.

So that you understand that past, Ralph's death came this way. About thirty minutes after getting morphine for his foot pain, his call light came on again. I responded, and he told me that his head hurt. The nurse was busy, so I called the resident myself. She was upset and promised to be down after talking with the attending physician.

By the time she arrived a few minutes later, Ralph was unconscious. She used an instrument to look at the tiny capillaries his eyes, and I remember thinking, "I wonder if she's doing that because she doesn't know what else to do?" She and I were powerless to stop what was happening before our eyes.

About a minute later, the boy's father showed a keener eye than either of us. He noticed his son had become paralyzed on one side. Just after that, the boy had a seizure. We hit the code button, and there was the usual clatter and confusion as the code team arrived.

It was too late. A headache, a coma, a seizure and, the final indignity, the code team starting IVs and performing CPR as they transported him to the ICU. The last was an exercise in futility. Ralph died badly— all witnessed by his distraught father.

From that night on, I kept that terrible sequence of events in mind whenever I had to care for a dying child: "This is bad, but not as bad as it might be."

There was another kind of death to which I was sometimes a belated witness. Because I was the only male nursing staff on nights, the shift supervisor would sometimes get me to help her with a larger child who'd died elsewhere. It was a somber journey using a special cart with a well like a bathtub. I'd pick up a shrouded but still warm child and place him or her in the tub. The supervisor would pull a sheet over the cart. Because the child was in the tub, the sheet lay flat, making it look like we were pushing an empty cart. The meaning of a body covered by a sheet would have been all too obvious. We'd take an elevator to the hospital's morgue, where I'd lift and place the child in a cooler's slide-out tray. I never learned those children's stories, but their final journey is worth noting.

To close on a less somber note, I should say this. Thanks to better treatments, today's deaths from childhood leukemia can be so gentle, the nurse who counseled our parents gave special advice to those flying home with a dying child. "It's possible," she explained to them, "that your child may begin to die on the flight. If that happens, say nothing to the flight attendants. Although it makes no sense, they are often under orders to immediately divert the aircraft to the nearest airport and call for an ambulance. Instead, treat your child as if she has fallen asleep. Put a pillow behind her head and place a blanket around her. Talk to her as if she could still hear you. Then when the plane reaches your destination, carry her off in your arms as if she's merely sleeping."

Next, we look at the occasions when I floated to other parts of the hospital.

19. Like the Pied Piper

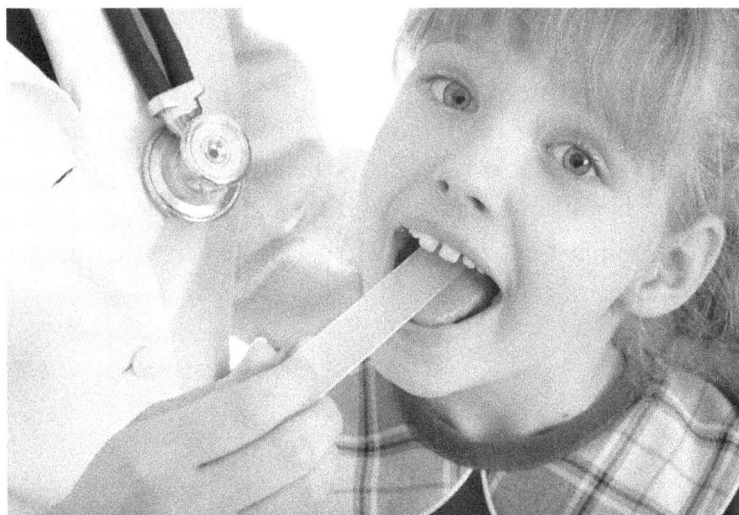

I didn't float that often when I worked nights on Hem-Onc. My expertise was more valuable there. But three nights out of every fourteen, the nursing student was working Hem-Onc, leaving me free. As a result, about once every six weeks, I'd be sent elsewhere in the hospital. Turn over among aides was high, particularly on nights, so I was soon one of the hospital's most experienced aides.

Surgery, one floor up, was perhaps the easiest assignment. If a surgery is done properly, there are no complications. The nurse might have pain medications to give, and I always had vital signs to check and the usual patient care like urinals. But in contrast to the stresses of Hem-Onc, nights on surgery were boring. I had trouble staying awake.

In contrast, floating to Babyland on the other side of the third-floor elevators left me anxious, although for no good reason. While we did occasionally take care of patients as young as three months on Hem-Onc, the tininess of my little Babyland charges alarmed me. Most patients on the medical unit were old enough to tell me what was wrong. These little babies could only cry mysteriously.

Fortunately, the wonderful nurses who worked there knew I was like a fish out of water and gave me their healthiest patients. At times that meant a night spent caring for four babies, each a graduate of the Neonatal ICU being fattened up before going home. Round and round, I went, the routine always the same. First, I'd do vital signs, then a bottle feed, a diaper change, and finally a little rocking to put them to sleep. Then it was on to the next baby. Nothing by the clock, just round and round endlessly. It was much like being a new parent.

My most unsettling float came when I was sent to Rehab, which was one floor down and cared for people with major disabilities. Because most were there for physical therapy during the day, one nurse was normally enough to watch over them as they slept. But that night the nurse had pointed out to the shift supervisor that she had two patients who were both dependent on respirators. If a problem arose with one, she wouldn't be able to watch the other. So that night I received my one and only experience carrying for people being kept alive by a machine. One I remember quite well.

Tanya was a twenty-one-year-old Asia woman who been in a diving accident that left her paralyzed from the neck down. She had some slight use of her arms, which she used to hold in place the tubing from the respirator that connected to the tracheotomy through which she breathed. She had no ability to breathe on her own. If that tubing popped loose, her breathing instantly stopped.

A family hardship brought her to us. Patients who can't move need to be turned once every two hours to prevent sores from developing. Her parents were exhausted from doing that every night. Tanya had come to test various machines to do the turning. That night, we were testing perhaps the most ridiculous of them, a bed that tilted from side to side. Every fifteen minutes, it'd shift to flat or tilted 45 degrees to the right or left. The absurdity came because, to keep her from falling to the floor, she had to be tightly strapped down. Those straps, I thought, were as likely to give her sores as lying in one position.

The event that unsettled me happened in the middle of the night when the nurse changed the clear plastic tubing to Tanya's respirator. The moment that tubing was disconnected, Tanya would stop breathing, so I got up in the bed and knelt alongside her. When the nurse disconnected the respirator tubing, I connected a Hope bag. That's a black rubber bag about the size and shape of a small loaf of bread. When I compressed it, Tanya's lungs filled with air. When I let up, her lungs deflated. For about a minute, she needed me to breathe. Every moment of her life, her ability to breathe depended on others. For a guy who values his independence above all else, that was upsetting.

A much lighter note sometimes came as I finished up night shift and got a call to report to Admissions and take children to day surgery on the fourth floor. Typically, these were small children who were getting either 'tubes' to deal with repeated ear infections or a tonsillectomy for chronic throat infections. They'd come in the morning with their parents and return home that afternoon. Day-only made their surgery cheaper and less emotionally traumatic.

Transporting those kids was sheer fun. When I arrived at Admissions, the kids would be waiting, their parents having already departed. They were told to follow me and off we'd go, typically with six to eight little ones following close at my heels, their eyes wide with wonder. I'd turn around every few seconds and count to make sure I wasn't losing any of my young charges. I felt like the Pied Piper of Hamelin.

Later, when I worked days on the teen unit, I saw day surgery from the other end. One day the anesthesiologists apparently over did putting the kids to sleep. When shift change rolled around that afternoon, the staffing for the post-op area was supposed to drop to a single nurse. But that day some five children were still asleep, so the nurse demanded extra help. I was sent to assist.

The post-op protocol for day surgery was short and simple. To go home, these children need only wake up, show acceptable vital signs, and void a single time.

After about an hour, we were left with only a two-year-old boy who wasn't waking up. At my insistence, a nurse anesthesiologist was called in and she pronounced him fine. The nurse and I then tried to fudge the rules. If we could only get him to void, we reasoned, we could pretend he was awake and send him home. We tried every trick we knew. We placed him on a toilet, gently shook him, and urged him to go. Nothing. We ran water. Nothing again. We even placed his hands in warm water, an old folk idea. Still nothing. At that point, the nurse decided she could manage alone, so I left.

Next, we return to Hem-Onc to look at my youngest patient and her fast IV.

20. Shana's Fast IV

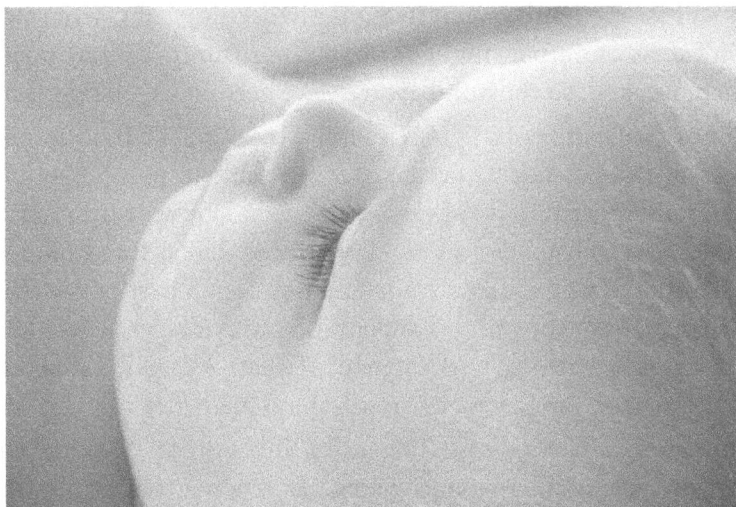

Ilooked at the tiny baby and back again to the number on the IV pump. "A hundred cc's an hour is way too much," I thought. "That's a rate for someone in their early teens." I spun around and headed for the nurse.

I'd been off when Shana had been admitted a couple of days before. At just three-months of age, she was the youngest leukemia patient I'd have. No, the nurse told me, that fast IV wasn't a mistake. A baby's kidneys don't concentrate waste well, so it had to run that fast to give the little girl enough fluid to clear out her just-finished chemotherapy. The nurse also told me that was why the baby wasn't wearing a diaper but instead slept face-down on one that was folded open. That made it easier to replace her constantly soggy diapers without waking her.

Of course, my alarm at that fast rate made sense. It meant Shana was getting her body weight in fluid about every five days, roughly equivalent to you or I getting a full gallon of fluids—over four large liter IV bags—pumped into our veins every day. That rate meant we needed to watch her carefully, which was why orders called for me to check her blood pressure every two hours.

But by now I was showing a streak of independence. Not satisfied following orders like a robot, I felt I should do more—in this case much more. An elevated blood pressure might come too late, happening only when there was no other place for all that fluid pouring into her to go. Medical guides gave other signs of fluid overload. Babies are usually chubby, so swelling in the hands and feet wouldn't be obvious. Breathing difficulties are hard to spot in a quietly sleeping baby. Charted fluid input in excess of output might work, but our tummy-on-an-open-diaper scheme leaked, so the numbers we were getting weren't perfect.

The best indication, the guides said, were signs of fluid pooling in her lungs as the left side of her heart wasn't able to pump blood out to her little fluid-stuffed body as fast as the right side sent it to her lungs. The guides said to listen for a 'crackling' sound, but at that time I wasn't sure what that meant. Lung sounds had not been a part of my training. So I decided that every time I replaced Shana's diaper, I would listen to her breathing with my stethoscope. If that changed, I'd sound the alarm. It wasn't in my orders, but it was good medicine.

Fortunately, I never heard that crackling sound. Looking back, I wonder why recognizing sounds weren't as much a part of my training as taking blood pressure. My search for indications other than blood pressure hints that by that time I was moving away from a focus on simply generating numbers for those yellow-jacketed flow sheets. I'd begun looking for other and often more subtle indications that one of my frail little patients might be in trouble. Like Sherlock Holmes at the scene of a crime, I wanted to spot every clue, however slight and ambiguous.

A medical seminar I attended offered more motivation. One of the perks of my job was attending for free any conference held at the hospital. What a physician might pay hundreds of dollars to attend, I could join for nothing. Of course, that also meant I needed to stay awake during the day when my body screamed for sleep. But getting better at what I did was worth a little misery.

One doctor intrigued me when he dealt with a problem that physicians regularly face. When a mother comes in, worried that her son or daughter has a serious infection, how does a family doctor or an ER physician decide if the child should be sent home or hospitalized? The latter is expensive for the parents and traumatic for the child, so it should not be done without a good reason. That, I realized, was exactly the judgment I must make with my kids. When should I suspect one was in serious trouble? When was the right time to raise an alarm?

The speaker that day had an answer. He'd examined research that explored every diagnostic tool a doctor might use when a child has an infection: tests like body temperature, white count, and blood sedimentation rate. All those, he said, came up lacking. The only reliable criteria was subjective. A child who, despite his sickness, was alert and aware of his surroundings, was likely to do well at home. One that seemed tired, listless and lethargic probably needed hospitalization.

I liked that, because it fitted with what I was discovering. My efforts to know these children and watch them like hawks now had another criteria. Were they tired, listless, unaware, or simply acting unusual either for themselves or for a typical child getting chemotherapy?

Of course, numbers still mattered, and I wasn't discarding them. Checking temperatures and alerting nurses when a kid spiked a temperature remained one of my most common activities. But I'd learned something vital caring for these children. I would be looking at more than the numbers to understand a child. I'd examine the whole picture and draw on my growing experience.

Now for a tragedy that was much too common on Hem-Onc. Despite all the fluids we were pumping into Shana, our youngest patient came through her first round of chemotherapy well, but she continued to retain a high risk for relapse. Leukemia treatment works best with children close to the most common age for the disease, which is about four years old. It doesn't work as well for those younger or older. In Shana's case, her diagnosis came so soon after birth, her doctors suspected she'd developed leukemia in the womb.

About nine months after the first night I cared for Shana, I remember going into her room and hearing the now cute little one-year-old say "Hi" to her mother's delight. She was learning to speak and might soon begin walking. Sadly, that was not to be. A few weeks later she died.

Helped by money from a distant and otherwise uninvolved father, Shana's mother was able to stay with her daughter during her entire hospital stay. That wasn't always the case. One of my saddest patients was a little girl who was left all alone as she lay dying. She's next.

21. LONELY SUSIE

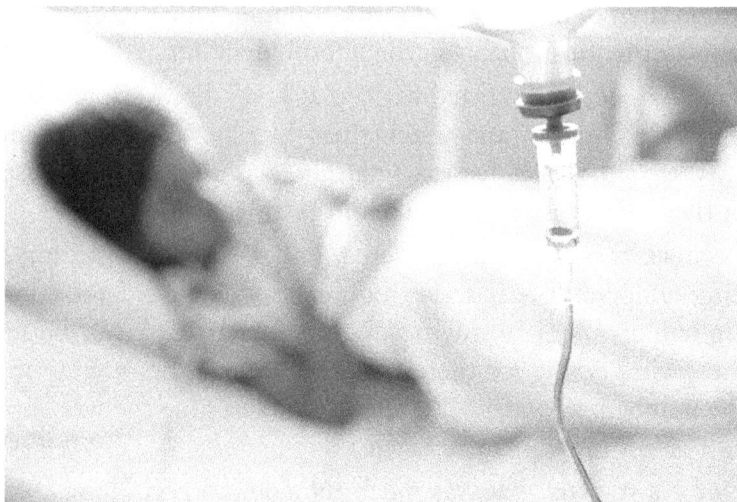

The trouble began with a short sentence I'd written in the girl's flow sheets: "This girl needs someone to stay with her at night." A day nurse with a nasty bent spotted it and informed the head nurse, who was Most Unhappy with me. That wasn't the proper thing to put in nursing notes, she told me sternly.

I said nothing, but I wasn't repentant. This girl did need someone to stay with her overnight. Where else was I going to write that? Should I scrawl it on the walls like graffiti?

Looking back, I wish I'd made more trouble, raising such a fuss that some kind soul would have been found to befriended this lonely little girl during in her last weeks on earth. Perhaps I should have even placed a longer and more strongly worded note in her medical chart, where usually only physicians made comments. That would have been even more Not Done, but might have brought results. After all, Susie's doctors bore the ultimate responsibility for her care.

Instead, hers was one of the saddest deaths I saw. To die young is bad. To die young and completely alone is infinitely worse. The fact that some nurses on the unit had hearts of stone shouldn't have deterred me. I should have done whatever it took to get her help.

Now for the details. Susie, so slender and small, was about eight years old, black, and almost certainly from a badly fractured family. She had the sad, woeful personality of someone who's learned through bitter experience to expect little from life, and life had certainly dealt badly with her. Medical attention came too late. She had a tumor in her upper chest that had so wrapped itself around her windpipe and the arteries to her heart, that surgery was impossible. Attempting to cut it out might have killed her. But worst of all was her loneliness. At her age, she must have been in some household, but no one there either cared enough to visit or, if they did care, had enough emotional strength to come.

Though their personalities differ greatly—solemn and sad versus impish and devious—Susie was a bit like Topsy, the little slave girl of about her age in Harriet Beecher Stowe's anti-slavery classic, *Uncle Tom's Cabin*. In the novel, Topsy had this fascinating conversation with the plantation's visiting New England spinster, Miss Ophelia:

"How old are you, Topsy?"

"Dun no, Missis," said the image, with a grin that showed all her teeth.

"Don't know how old you are? Didn't anybody ever tell you? Who was your mother?"

"Never had none!" said the child, with another grin.

"Never had any mother? What do you mean? Where were you born?"

"Never was born!," persisted Topsy, with another grin, that looked so goblin-like, that, if Miss Ophelia had been at all nervous, she might have fancied that she had got hold of some sooty gnome from the land of Diablerie; but Miss Ophelia was not nervous, but plain and business-like, and she said, with some sternness,

"You mustn't answer me in that way, child; I'm not playing with you. Tell me where you were born, and who your father and mother were."

"Never was born," reiterated the creature, more emphatically; "never had no father nor mother, nor nothin'. I was raised by a speculator, with lots of others. Old Aunt Sue used to take car[e] on us."

Susie was in a similar situation. Her lack of visitors gave the appearance that she "never had no father nor mother, nor nothin.'" As far as I knew, no one apart from hospital staff spent time with her during her last weeks except once, when a tall, respectable, middle-age black woman carrying a large Bible spent the night. We were told she was an aunt, but I suspect that was an honorary title. She might have been a kindly soul with distant ties to the girl's absent family.

My frustration came because there was no way I could provide Susie with the attention she needed. With great effort I could squeeze out 45 minutes just after midnight to rock Eli to sleep. He was young and, once asleep, stayed asleep. I did rock Susie to sleep each night. But she was older and had such a terrifying storm raging inside her that she couldn't stay asleep. There was no way I could find time to help her to fall asleep again and again. My frustration about that explains my most medically incorrect note. My failure to get something done still infuriates me.

Often when a system fails as badly as ours did with Susie, someone intervenes to make up for at least some of its deficiencies. That's what happened with her. Near the end, it became clear that she would die when the growing tumor crushed her windpipe, making it impossible for her to breathe. To prepare for that, she was put on IV morphine, which would remove any discomfort from a lack of oxygen.

Fortunately, as Susie's breathing became difficult, a nurse—the same nurse I later describe as questioning me about Jackie's death—stayed over, held her, and talked to her as she breathed her last. Susie's last weeks were far more lonely than they should have been, but she at least she wasn't alone at her death, thanks to the kindness of that nurse.

Since then, I've wondered what might be done for children in situations such as hers. Organizations such as Make a Wish give children one final happy experience and that's good. But one happy experience doesn't make up for a lonely death. And unfortunately, the expectations of someone like Susie are so low, I'm not sure she'd have an answer if you'd asked her, "What would you like most to do?"

I can only speculate about how such an organization would work. It'd need to be built around highly dedicated volunteers who could devote many hours when necessary. In Susie's case, that meant staying overnight every night for weeks and getting little sleep. It might also mean being with her at least part of each day. Short trips to a park or zoo were possible, since there was no medical treatment to interrupt. And if by happenstance she died in a sunny park with her new friend, that would be far better than dying all alone in a hospital bed.

My Nights with Leukemia

It'd also be important that the two—the child and her friend—somehow got on with one another. Years ago I visited a young man who'd been in the hospital for some eight years following a motorcycle accident that'd left him paralyzed from the neck down. Even though I came once a week for several months, nothing happened between us. The visits stayed stiff and formal. That's not what we want for these kids.

On the other hand, the little Jackie I discuss later and I hit it off from the start. Something did click between us. Although I could do little to help that man through a boring hour in Dallas's Parkland Hospital, I did help Jackie through many a tough night. Friendships can be arranged, but they can't be contrived or forced.

So something would need to click between child and volunteer or the adult's well-meant visiting might only irritate an already troubled child. Perhaps the process could begin with several visitors who'd come to read stories or play games with these kids. That'd allow the child to select a friend. Little Jackie, for instance, seems to have appreciated my feeble attempts to sing her to sleep.

For older children, reading stories might be better. A six-year-old boy might like an "Uncle Bob" who reads boy stories such as *Treasure Island* to him. In any case, the relationship shouldn't be forced. It should develop naturally. That's certainly far better than the alternative—sad kids dying all alone. I saw three such cases during my twenty-six months at this hospital. That was three too many.

And no, the two friends need not be alike. Sometimes differences attract. Later, I discuss an unlikely friendship between two girls on the teen unit. Tina was tiny, frail, shy, and dying of a brain tumor. Hanna was several years older, large, robust, and outgoing. Hanna's freely chosen friendship with the dying Tina is one of the bravest acts I've ever seen. More later.

Next we'll look at Roger, a boy who, although he was in no danger of dying, had been abandoned at our hospital and all but forgotten.

22. ROGER, BORN TOO SOON

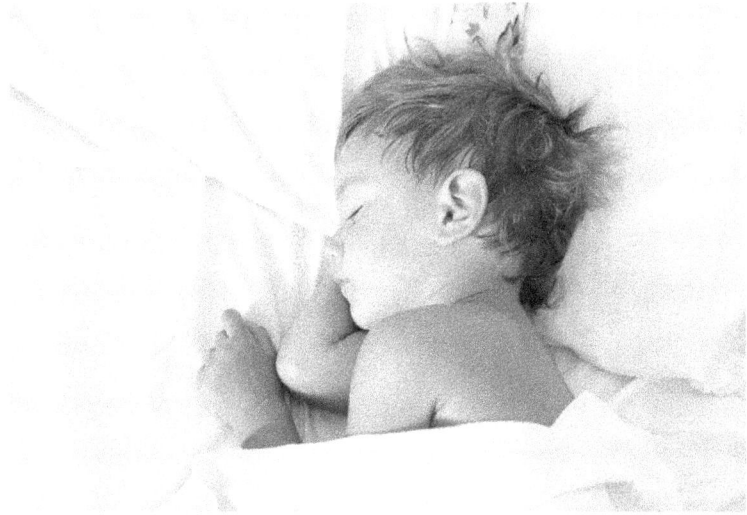

Sometimes the leading edge of medicine becomes the bleeding edge. Progress has costs, and Roger's condition, I was told, had been one of those costs. Born prematurely, the respirator that kept him alive also left his lungs scarred with what was then called hyaline membrane disease. Today, we know how to prevent it, but that knowledge came too late for him. Roger was born too soon in a double sense.

Since his birth, he had been the victim of a system that was poorly suited for his situation. His prematurity meant a long hospitalization that broke what must have already been fragile ties to his parents. As far as I know, no one in his family visited him. Now about three years old, he didn't need to be in a hospital. The air around us is about 21 percent oxygen. He needed a little more than that but not much. He did quite well with a 24 percent supply.

Roger's real problem was social. He was surrounded by a sea of continually changing faces. The nursing staff came and went every eight hours. The kids in his room changed every few days. Every few months brought new nursing staff. The result was a boy with no attachments to people—a boy learning to tune out his human surroundings. I still have a picture of him curled up and sleeping in his crib. He looks disturbingly like a caged animal.

The only member of our staff he gave any attention was a cheerful housekeeper who made a big show of talking with him each morning. Housekeeping staff turned over slowly, so she may have been the only person he had seen regularly throughout his life. Obviously, his situation was not good. What had been an ordinary baby born early was becoming a seriously troubled youth with no interest in people.

A couple of years later, I'd volunteer at a university's child research center, working with children who had severe behavior disorders, mostly autism. One I've already mentioned was Rita, a little girl of about four, who'd been raised by an insane grandmother who kept her locked in a closet. Like Roger, she knew little about relating to people, but she was desperate to enter our world. When I greeted her each morning, she wanted to be hugged and struggled desperately to talk.

Unfortunately, Roger wasn't interested in hugs or conversations. For him, we were mere background. He would not look at me unless I deliberately moved into his line of sight, and then he would glance away. Almost all his life had been spent in a drab four-bed ward. No visits to the zoo, no stories read, no playing in the park, and no Christmas with grandparents. Nothing but that same room, that same crib, and a constantly changing stream of faces.

Unfortunately, as staff we had little incentive change his situation. His presence made our work easier. He took up a bed in a room with three other kids. If he left, the string of children who would replaced him would require more time and attention. That's why it was easy not to say: "Hey, we need to do something about this kid. He is getting weird, really weird."

Our inattention to Roger's need for a home and parents went beyond the nursing staff. The root problem was that he wasn't a typical patient. Hospitals usually deal with kids whose parents want to take them home as soon as possible. They aren't accustomed to having a child who's abandoned without being first neglected or abused. Finding a foster home or adoptive parents required thinking outside the box.

Fortunately, that happened. Adoptive parents were found. A Lutheran minister and his wife adopted our odd little Roger, giving him the love he needed. Roger left us long after he should, but hopefully in time to get back on track. That's what I heard happened. He was even weaned off oxygen. All that took was getting him moving around like other boys his age.

As I look back, Roger's stay illustrates my greatest unhappiness with myself during this time. Around me were problems needing correcting, some heart-rending. Yes, those problems weren't in my job description. I was an aide, so not much was. But that didn't meant I shouldn't have acted, even if all I did was point out a bad situation to others. We should never forget, wherever we are, that we are our brother's keeper. That's especially true when these brothers and sisters are abandoned, frightened, sick, or even weird kids like Roger.

In Roger's case, the politics were easy. There was no downside to directing attention at him. The hospital was spending a considerable sum of money having him warm a mattress. That was because it felt responsible for his disability. But if a good home could be found, that money could go to other needy children.

But what, you may ask, about situations where there's a considerable risk to calling for change? Doing the right thing isn't always safe or easy. Sometimes change costs money. Sometimes it embarrasses well-placed people. At other times it challenges what George Orwell once called the "smelly little orthodoxies" that haunt every institution and every profession. Medicine is not immune to that affliction. A few guidelines may help if you find yourself in a situation where change is needed but opposition is possible.

1. **Make sure your motives are good.** Orwell used "smelly little orthodoxies" to described what Charles Dickens fought against with his novels. Dickens, he wrote, was "a man who is always fighting against something, but who fights in the open and is not frightened, the face of a man who is generously angry." Dickens, Orwell wrote, fought out of a genuine anger at some evil, but without "malignity" or a desire to "triumph." Advocating change should never be an underhanded way to crush those we dislike or to make ourselves look superior. We should be "generously angry," even wishing our opponents to change. For an example, think of Scrooge in Dicken's masterpiece, *A Christmas Carol.*

2. **Don't focus on yourself.** It helps if we're not worried about getting the credit. Over a couple of night shifts, I saw two cases where a connector for IV lines separated from the tubing itself, and I heard about a third. Those didn't seem isolated incidents. The lines, I decided, must be defective. But rather than go down to the nursing office and report the problem, I ran an experiment. I slipped the idea into conversations with nurses, hoping one would raise the issue. I'm not sure I was the

cause—after all each of those cases had triggered an incident report—but the next day word came down. Our latest shipment of IV tubing had been defective, it said, so we would be using older tubing until it was replaced. As President Harry Truman said, "It is amazing how much you can accomplish when it doesn't matter who gets the credit." Do good, but don't insist on getting the praise.

3. **Prepare in advance.** Yes, some situations may not give you time for thought and reflection. Sometimes you must speak out before you can come up with good arguments. That was my situation (described later) when I had only seconds to come up with a reason to persuade a resident to order a blood chemistry test on Brian. But in most cases, you'll have time to develop reasons. In the case of weird little Roger, he wasn't in any immediate danger. I could have honed my arguments over several weeks and gotten advice from nurses and social workers. Speed wasn't important. Acting was.

4. **Consider who to approach.** In most organizations there are people who're the best positioned and most likely to help your cause. Contact them rather than someone who's more resistant. When I complained in those nursing notes about little Susie needing someone to stay with her at night, those who read it—an ill-tempered day nurse and an overly critical head nurse—weren't the best people to see what I'd written. The first lacked heart, while the second's head was filled with rules. The nurse who cared for the social and emotional needs of families would have been a better choice, particularly since she might not know about the trouble Susie was having with sleep. Learn from my mistake and think through who's the best person to tell. It'll make a big difference.

5. **Be aware of politics.** Realize that there may be special interests who aren't be happy with what you're suggesting. Hospitals are prone to turf wars and pecking orders. You can't always avoid those conflicts, but you can prepare and enter with your eyes open.

6. **Choose your words carefully.** Several years ago, I had a job filtering people into special events such as weddings and memorial services with someone who also worked at a funeral home. Both are situations where people are easily offended, and I noticed that she carefully chose the words she used. Rather than say, "You can't go in here. You must go around the building," she'd say, "The family has asked that you...." Remember the four Ws—Well-chosen Words Work Wonders.

7. **Realize that there may be costs.** Not all suggestions are well received. Some may get you into trouble, and a few many even put your career in jeopardy. In that respect, I had it easy. I hadn't made a major investment of time and money to get my job and wasn't pursuing a career in nursing or medicine. If I were badly treated, I could walk out. Most doctors and nurses have less freedom. They've spent years getting where they are now. Gaining a reputation as a troublemaker, however unfair, might leave them unable to do what they've trained for so long to do. That doesn't mean you shouldn't act. After all, lives may hang in the balance. Just carefully count the cost first.

8. **Find allies.** When someone powerful takes offense, you must protect yourself. Try to win someone equally powerful to your side. Recall when I described that housekeeper who took on two doctors for not following isolation rules. Her position was improved when one doctor took her side. It helps to have friends in high places or, failing that, at least someone who is willing to speak up for you, so you're not alone.

9. **Stay balanced.** Whatever happens, don't let conflict wreck your relationship with those around you or destroy your ability to work effectively. As much as is possible, don't personalize conflicts. Stay calm and agree to disagree.

10. **Retain your perspective.** Shortly before I entered graduate school, a budget crunch almost led the medical school to eliminate the medical history and ethics department where I'd study. One day, when the department head was away, his secretary took me into his office and pointed to a picture placed so only he could see it. It showed him as a young Marine fighting on a mountainous, Japanese-held island in the Pacific. The struggle for that island was long and bitter, with thousands of casualties on both sides. As he fought to save his department, she said, he'd look at that picture and remind himself that the present wasn't as bad as that. Find similar ways to keep your spirits up when things get tough. Often the best way is to get your thoughts off yourself and put them on *why* you're fighting and *who* you're fighting for.

Next, we look at funerals and how the hospital staff I worked with responded to them.

My Nights with Leukemia

23. Families and Funerals

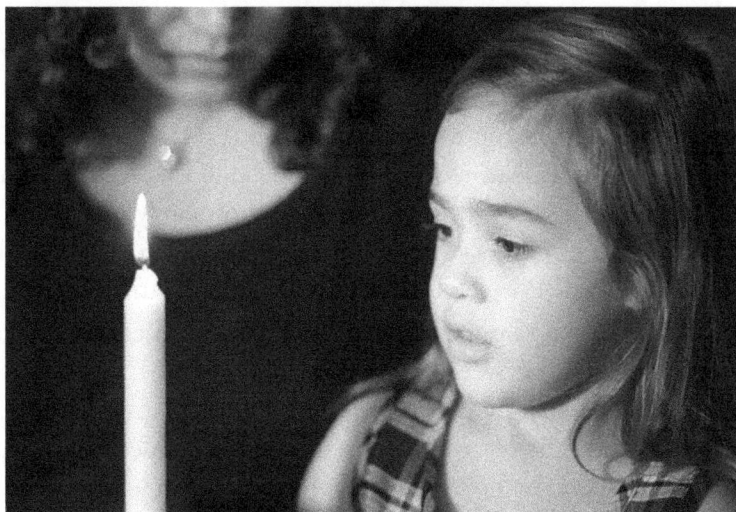

Funerals usually follow deaths. For some of the children we'd been treating, the family would invite the hospital's staff to attend either a funeral or memorial service. As I wrestled with this book, I tried to see patterns in those invitations, as well as why I and others went. Here's what I've come up with.

For Eli—the first child I cared for who died—there apparently wasn't an invitation. I certainly don't remember one. His mother, so overwhelmed by her child's sickness, must have also been so overcome by his death, that she didn't have the resources for anything more than the simplest of funerals. To be able to give to others, you must have something to give. She had nothing left. Some parents were too overwhelmed to plan a funeral to which staff could be invited.

Sadder by far were situations where no one in a child's family seemed to care. For those children, I suspect there wasn't much, if any, of a service. It's hard to imagine a child who got so little attention while dying getting much afterward.

Susie, the little girl with the chest tumor who was left all alone, might not have even had a funeral. I don't know. Perhaps there was a pauper's burial, paid for by the state and handled as a charity by a church or funeral home. Yes, I should have tried to find out, but it was all too easy to be distracted. There were always sick children, and some were always dying. Besides, by the time she died, I'd transferred to working days with teens, so she was no longer my patient. Excuses.

For other children, although they were clearly loved by their families, there simply hadn't been enough time for the staff to establish a relationship. I doubt I spoke more than a few dozen words with Ralph, the boy who suffered a brain hemorrhage and died a few hours after he was admitted. The same was true of Tammy, a chatty teen-aged girl with Down syndrome that we'll discuss later. She was admitted one afternoon and died the following morning, also probably of a brain hemorrhage. We were strangers when we met, and remained strangers hours later when they died. People don't usually attend a stranger's funeral.

In other cases, the reason was emotional. Sometimes, no special relationship developed between a child or parents and the nursing staff. The contact stayed strictly professional. Kindness is giving and can be one way. Friendship, even between an adult and child, is an exchange. Kids such as Binky, the boy that God made, were able to reach out in friendship and received friendship in return. But there were other kids who seemed too withdrawn to reach out—Susie and later Tina come to mind. They received kindness from staff, but there was never that mutual bond that leaves people needing to honor them at their death. For that, these children should not be blamed. It takes a special maturity to build relationships with adults at an early age, especially while dying.

In fact, as I look back on the funeral invitations that we received, one fact stands out clearly. All came from strong, two-parent families with enough emotional reserves to share their grief with others. That was particularly true of Binky, the boy that God made. His family took the time to arrange a special memorial service for those at the hospital who had cared for him and to have their pastor lead it. That was their thank you for all the care we'd given him.

That was also true of a girl that I've otherwise not mentioned. Her father was a chief petty officer on one of the nuclear submarines that operated out of what was then the Naval Submarine Base Bangor. During the Cold War, the base—one of our chief deterrents against a Soviet attack—maintained high levels of security. The family not only invited us to a memorial service at their home, they took care of the details of getting us clearance onto the base.

A strong and stable two-parent family was also characteristic of what was beyond doubt the most remarkable family I saw during my two years of caring for dying children. Sociologists would reduce this dad, mom, and son to a mere blue collar family, as if income or employment defines someone. (I recall him being a car mechanic.) Cynics and snobs would have gone further and sneered at them as "rednecks," laughing at their ways, as if the entire world is—or at least ought to be—like those who live in the tiny, affluent enclaves of a few large coastal cities.

This couple was actually strong and resourceful, unafraid to tackle any problem that arose. It was their can-do spirit that impressed me and reminded me of those who settled our nation's frontiers. All too many Americans have lost touch with death, fearing it and delegating it to professionals. Thanks to advances in public health and medicine, they've particularly lost touch with the deaths of children. It's good that we have to deal with that so rarely, but unfortunate that we no longer know how. This family was not like that. They were rooted in an older tradition, one in which the deaths of children were still common, and one in which families still managed all aspects of dying.

Their only child, Frankie, was a quiet but friendly five-year-old boy with an inoperable brain tumor. While he was in the hospital, his parents were deeply involved in his care. Most intriguing for me was the fact they showed no deference to a hospital's formal, hierarchical, professional-versus-lay structure. Theirs was a culture in which any relationship quickly became personal. They wanted to know you, and they wanted you to know them. Think of television shows such as *Little House on the Prairie* or *The Waltons*. That was their world, and it was an appealing one.

When it became obvious that our hospital could do nothing more for Frankie, his parents took him home to handle his final care themselves, after getting the necessary training from our nurses. That's when something surprising happened. After he died, they drove several hours and even took a ferry to bring his body to us for a possible autopsy. They arrived late one evening and invited the staff on duty that night—me included—to come to the ER to view his body. They assumed, as a matter of course, that the people who had cared for him while he was alive would want to see him after he died. Medicine, for all its complexities, did not intimidate them in the least. No problem was too great to be faced. No difficulty could not be overcome. Even death held no fear.

That evening, Frankie's father told me about his boy's last month, which was spent in a coma. Feeding wasn't a problem. We'd taught the couple how to insert an NG tube and give formula. When his brain tumor caused him to stop breathing, they would perform mouth-to-mouth resuscitation for a few minutes until he began to breath again. Finally, the day came when he did not breath on his own. His tumor had grown too large. The father and mother agreed that they would continue mouth-to-mouth resuscitation for forty-five more minutes. If he didn't breathe after that, they would let him go.

As you might expect, we were invited to Frankie's funeral. There, the family's strength and resourcefulness were again obvious. They wanted to have an open-casket funeral, but the funeral home where they planned to hold the service didn't have refrigeration. So the father worked out an arrangement for storage at another funeral home, taking care of the transportation himself. That close and intimate involvement was their way of expressing love for their son. Allowing us to be part of the funeral, including that open casket, was their way of thanking us.

At this point, I won't mince words. Those who mock that family's behavior are the ones who're out of touch. In doing what they did for their son, both before and after his death, these parents showed a wisdom that's as old as the hills. Here's why.

Losing any child that had been my patient left a hole, large or small, in me. For weeks or even months I'd been caring for that child. Now he or she was gone. That's something you expect with older relatives. It's not something you expect with a child. No matter how long anticipated, it was hard to accept. It didn't seem normal. It didn't seem right.

In fact, as I look back over all the children who died, there's a clear division between those who died on my shift and those who died at other times and places. When children died under my care, they really did die. I was part of what happened. Typically, I was in the room when they stopped breathing, or I saw their body just afterward. In some cases, I even prepared them for the morgue, washing and wrapping them in a plastic shroud. That eased my sense of loss. One part of me wasn't denying what another knew to be true. I had closure.

For those who died when I wasn't there, the experience was different. A part of me refused to accept what had happened. I had cared for them one night, talking with them and bringing them what they wanted. The next night they were gone, with someone else now in their room. How was that different from when they went home well? It wasn't—or at least it didn't feel like it was.

Of course, if a child died at the hospital, the evening nurse would tell us about it. But those were mere words, little different from reading an obituary notice. My conscious, reasoning mind knew this child was dead, but something deep inside remained in denial. The result was that hole. A child who should be there wasn't.

That's why traditional rituals matter. They give us a structure in which to let someone go. Going to a funeral substitutes for not being present when they died. That's why I and others on the nursing staff often found ourselves wanting to attend, whatever the complications. What we felt is a intrinsic to being human. That's why evidence of funerals extends back into our most remotest prehistory. Ancient graves from tens of thousands of years ago had flowers in them. Long ago, people missed the beauty others brought to their lives—hence the lovely flowers.

When I attended a child's funeral, I had completion. I knew they were really gone. I could write "Finished" to their story, brief as it was. If that were true for me, merely an aide caring for them their last few months, imagine what it must have meant for those close to them, particularly those who'd known them all their lives. A funeral matters.

Of course, not everyone at the hospital attended funerals. I sometimes wonder what it must have been like for our talented doctors when their young patients died despite their best efforts. With a disease like leukemia, at the very end there was usually little need for their skills. Our nurses knew how to care for a dying child and often made the necessary decisions for themselves. Their attitude was, 'The doctors have done what they could and failed. We'll take over from here."

I also had a role. In some cases, when the final care was uncomplicated and nursing demands from other children great, the responsibility for final care fell almost exclusively on me. In those situations, the physicians became superfluous, to be called for only when the death certificate needed completing, as I noted with Charlie, the boy with *cri du chat*. Unlike the nursing staff, doctors were rarely part of the dying process and were almost never there when a child died. They had no chance for closure. "Did they need it?," I wondered.

What about funerals? These physicians could find closure there, so that's why their absence always struck me as worthy of note. I'm sure that in small towns physicians do attend the funerals of patients. The patient would have also been a friend and neighbor. But I never saw a physician at any of the children's funerals I attended. I know they are busy people with heavy demands on their time, so I'm not saying they *should* be there. I'm merely wondering what impact that absence had on them. Did they miss these children or had they adopted a professional detachment that rendered them immune from the pangs felt by others. To this day I don't know.

Yes, I also realize that for a physician who has spent years honing their skills in a particular specialty, the risk of burnout holds far more terror than for nurses, much less for me. If they find themselves unable to render care, what could they do? Could they discard those long years of training? I comment more on that in *Hospital Gowns* in a chapter called "Understanding Doctors." You might want to read it.

Remember too that when nurses find themselves crushed by the grief of providing one type of care, they can move on to something quite different and perhaps less emotionally draining. I've seen that happen with friends who are nurses. I had even more freedom, so I could take more risks. Having invested little in formal training, I could leave medicine at any time.

Next we'll look at something that's less emotional and more medical. The Hem-Onc unit where I worked was one of the first in the world to do bone marrow transplants on children.

24. Life in the Blood

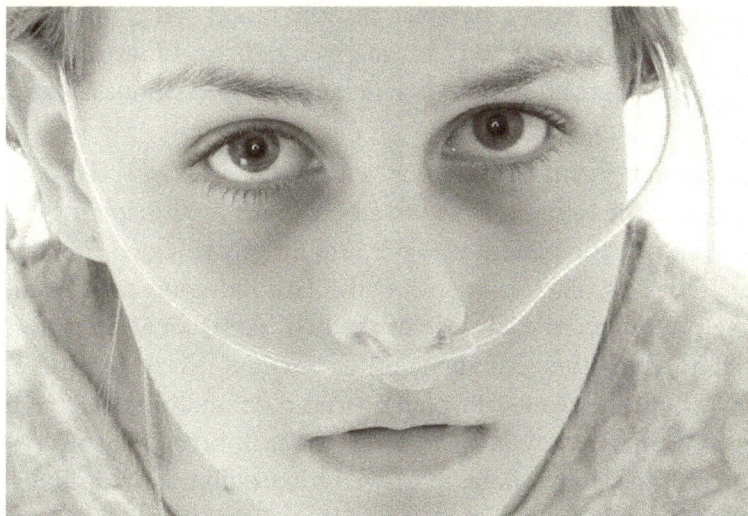

At the time I was involved in treating childhood leukemia, we had almost no other options once our basic course of treatment with Methotrexate (sometimes supplemented with radiation) was exhausted. The only exception was a bone marrow transplant. At that time, bone marrow transplants were new and rare. I was told that a large cancer research center a few miles away oversaw some half the transplants in the entire world. We worked with them, handling bone marrow transplants for children and teens. My first experience was a fourteen-year-old boy I took care of shortly after I began work on Hem-Onc.

There were several reasons why these transplants were rare. One was the extremely high dose of full-body radiation given. When I mentioned to a friend who worked in radiation medicine that the boy I was caring for had just received a 600 REM, full-body dose, she turned to me and said with shock, "That's a lethal dose." "Yes," I said, "that's the first stage in our treatment. We give them enough radiation to kill them."

It was. Radiation exposure is lethal at many levels. Lower dosages don't kill quickly. Instead, they increase the risk for acquiring cancer later in life. That's what has happened with many of the survivors of Hiroshima and Nagasaki.

Higher doses, those in the range we were using, kill much more quickly, usually within a few weeks. They destroy the rapidly multiplying cells necessary for life, particularly those in the blood. That's why radiation works with leukemia. It kills the cells that are multiplying out of control. Of course, like our chemotherapy, that lethal dose was a blunt instrument. It also kills a patient's healthy blood cells, hence the need for a bone marrow transplant. Those given radiation must get new, leukemia-free blood marrow from a matched donor. Without it, they'll die. That's what the transplant is.

Unlike other forms of radiation treatment, no great precision is required to give the radiation used in a bone marrow transplant. As it was described to me, the patient was put into heavily shielded room and everyone else leaves. Then two powerful cobalt radiation sources come up from the floor, one on each side of the bed. After an allotted time, the sources return to storage and the others reenter. That's because a peculiarity of a bone-marrow transplant is that the radiation needs to be given over a patient's entire body in order to reach blood cells everywhere, particularly those in the bone marrow. Other radiation treatments are as narrowly focused as possible, so radiation sources designed to target one organ won't work over an entire body. That was one reason why so few centers did bone marrow transplants at that time. It required an expensive radiation tool that most cancer centers did not have.

The second reason for the scarcity of transplants came after that lethal dose. No, it wasn't a surgery. For the person receiving a bone marrow transplant, the procedure is trivial. It's like a blood transfusion. I did several myself. The nurse hung the bag with the filtered bone marrow, diluted with a saline solution, and started the infusion. I then monitored for complications while it dripped into the patient. That's all.

In a sense, it was even easier than a transfusion. Since the blood in a bone marrow transplant must be much more closely matched, the chance of a sudden reaction was almost zero. Even if there had been a reaction, the transfusion would have had to continue. It was like a heart transplant. After a diseased heart is removed, the transplant must be put in. Without it, the patient dies.

For a bone marrow transplant, the real magic begins after the transfusion. The new bone marrow does the real work, settling down inside the bone marrow of its new host, where it grows, sending out healthy cells. That evil blood factory I wrote about earlier has been shut down and its machinery destroyed, replaced over several weeks by healthy new bone marrow.

My Nights with Leukemia

For the donor, a transplant was more complicated, but only a day surgery. At that time, I was told, the surgeons would drill into the hip bones and extract bone marrow. Because the blood match has to be close, back then the only donors were close relatives. When no relative was a match—it's a one-in-four chance for a brother or sister—no transplant was possible.

That was a third reason why transplants were rare. In many cases there was no matched donor. For a single night I cared for a teen-aged girl from Brazil who'd come with her uncle on the slight chance he'd be a match. Thousands of people in her country had responded to a television campaign to fund her trip. He wasn't a match, and she returned home to die. Very sad.

Matched donors are that important. A few years later, a bone marrow registry was set up to find unrelated donors. I immediately signed up, and I've been waiting for a call ever since. Please sign up through your local blood bank. You might be the only person who could save someone's life.

The aftermath of that transplant was the fourth and most important reason why so few hospitals did transplants. In the weeks afterward, the patient's blood counts would plummet as the blood cells that received the radiation died and the new, transplanted cells multiplied to replace them. The decline in red blood cells and platelets could be remedied by transfusions, but far less could be done for the white cells that fight infections. A normal white blood count is in between 4,000 and 10,000. I've taken care of children with counts as low as 100. As a result, there was a several week period during which patients were virtually without an immune system and dependent of a hospital's skill with isolation and antibiotics. Only top-tier hospitals have those skills.

The fifth reason bone marrow transplants were rare was the most depressing, particularly with children. Bone marrow transplants were a limited resource, with no open-to-all wait lists. Transplants were for those who had the proper connections and an ability to pay their high cost, a cost not usually covered by insurance since the treatment was still experimental. That left kids dependent on who their parents were.

As a result, many of the kids whose lives might have been saved by a transplant never got a chance. As best I could tell, for most of our children the option was never mentioned. It'd have been cruel to offer something only to say, "but you can't afford it" or even worse, "but there aren't enough places open." A nurse who worked at the cancer center pioneering bone marrow transplants told me that she'd taken careful note of her patients. There were many relatives of physicians, she said, but none from the families of plumbers such as her husband.

Before you condemn those doing these transplants, keep in mind the limitations imposed by finances. Taking in children whose parents could not pay would have strained the center's budget and limited the number of patients who could be treated, meaning that more rather than fewer children would die. The children who lived might have had richer parents, but there were still more of them. Also, keep in mind that the treatment was still experimental, meaning that the success rate was lower than it would be later after more experience had been gained.

Nor was success assured. One boy I cared for died—the only bone marrow transplant death I saw. That boy's death came from what's called graft-versus-host disease (GVHD). The bone marrow he'd received from his brother saw his body as foreign and attacked it. I saw the early signs when he complained when I put a probe under his arm to take his temperature. "That's not normal," I thought, but unfortunately I didn't pursue the thought any further. Only after GVHD was diagnosed a couple of days later did I remember that a sensitive skin or a rash is one early sign.

That same cancer center nurse also told me of a situation where a "rich Saudi oil sheik" whose son had leukemia approached the center with an offer. If he gave them one million dollars, enough at that time to care for ten children, would his son move to the front of the line? The doctors concluded that, with a million dollars to spend, they could quickly enlarge their program, so no other patient would suffer by being held back because that boy had jumped to the front of the line. The enlarged program could then treat more people. It you like to think about ethics, ponder that one. If no one else gets harmed, is providing special treatment to those with money acceptable?

Also, keep in mind that the costs associated with a bone marrow transplant have remained remarkably stable over the years—a tribute to the skills of the physicians and medical staff involved. When I worked with these children, parents were told than a transplant would cost about $100,000. Now, transplants for children with leukemia cost from $150,000 to $200,000. That's less than inflation in general, and far less than the rise is the costs of most medical care. Bone marrow transplants are becoming more affordable.

One reason for the limited rise in costs may be the absence of that great bane of good medical care—ambulance-chasing lawyers. The potential for lawsuits distorts care, adding to costs and pressuring doctors to treat in ways that look good in court but do nothing for patients. Fortunately, the fear of lawsuits has little impact on a treatment that offers a reasonable hope for those whose situation is otherwise hopeless. Families are more accepting when that one last chance fails.

This rise in the general availability of bone marrow transplants also illustrates that medicine does have a trickle-down effect. Over time, treatments that were available for only a select few become more routine, more readily available, and more often covered by insurance.

In fact, what happened with bone marrow transplants—a move from the top down—reverses a common pattern in medicine. I once heard a noted pediatric surgeon point out that, when heart surgery on children was new and risky, a disproportionate share of the first patients were children with Down Syndrome. However, he said with obvious disgust, once that surgery became safer—although still expensive—there was a period during which surgeries on children with Down became rare. Physicians took several years to realize that the very children who'd first received that life-saving surgery still deserved it.

In addition to caring for children who could only be cured with cutting-edge medicine, I also cared for children and teens who came to us simply to die. We look at that next.

25. Breathe Christy, Breathe

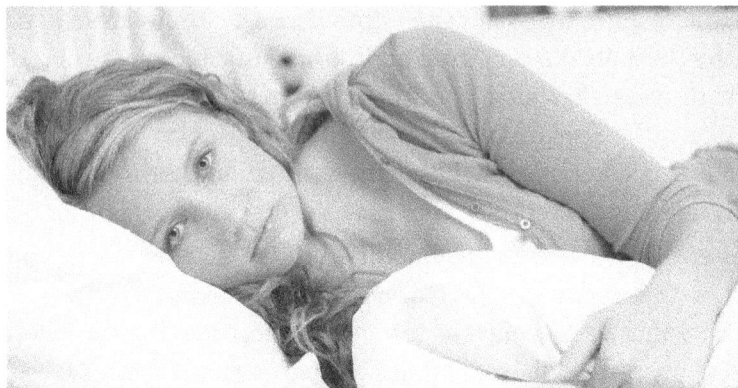

Working with dying children taught me something I'd not known before. Death is not simply a process that comes when it will like the falling of a stone from the face of a cliff. Even frail children can exercise an impressive amount of control over if, when, and how they die. Some who ought to die by all that medicine knows, refuse to give up and live. Others choose the place and time of their death. "Not now and here, but then and there," they say.

I've already mentioned Pauline, the little girl who refused to die at our hospital, but let herself pass away ten minutes after she reached home. That happens more often than we realize. Those who know American history can point to two of our nation's most esteemed founders, John Adams and Thomas Jefferson, who died on precisely the fiftieth anniversary of the Declaration of Independence. Read the accounts of their deaths, and you come away feeling that each was hanging on until that day—The Day—arrived. Each was also aware that only the two of them remained from that momentous event.

That's why one night during report when the evening nurse mentioned that our latest transfer would have her fifteenth birthday the following Thursday, the thought passed through my mind, "that's when she'll die." I was probably not the only one.

No, we didn't normally care for dying teens. At that time a teen unit existed to deal with the more complex emotional issues that surround them. You can read of my experiences there in *Hospital Gowns*.

Christy was an exception or, to be more accurate, Christy's mother was an exception. Most parents of dying children recognize that the nursing staff is doing all it can to ease the dying process. Christy's mom was not like that. She was angry that her daughter had an inoperable brain tumor and was directing her anger at the most readily available target—our nurses. She had wrecked her relationships with all the nurses on the teen unit, so the hospital had transferred her daughter to us. That mother's problems were now our problems. To be fair, I should mention that Christy was her only child, and that she was probably past the age of childbearing. She was losing the only child she would ever have. Her anger wasn't helping her daughter, but it had a reason.

Brain tumors can be silent, painless killers. No treatment was needed to ease Christy's death, so there was nothing for her nurses to do. Until the very last, when she lapsed into a coma and her care became more complicated, she was my patient. She was confined to a bed, able only to turn from side to side, so I dropped into her room as often as I could, talking and getting her anything she needed. Each night over the next week she became a little quieter and more withdrawn.

Then came the night that would usher in her birthday. When I arrived, she was in a coma. I finished my usual start-of-shift duties with the children and came into her room a little after midnight. "She is now fifteen," I told myself.

For unconscious patients, it was standard procedure to turn them every couple of hours to prevent bed sores, so that's what I did. Unfortunately, that shifted her now-shallow breathing from her left to her right lung. She stopped breathing.

Should I just let her die? She'd been classified "No Code," because a code response made no sense. It would trigger a chain of medical interventions that had no point. But her family wasn't there, and the medical orders did include a provision for 'blow by' oxygen. So, I gently shook her and said, "Breathe Christy, breathe." Then, as she began to breathe again, I placed an oxygen tube close to her face.

A call was made, and her mother arrived about half-an-hour later. That's when something wonderful happened. In the preceding week, the mother had done to our nurses what she done to those on the teen unit. She wrecked any good will they might feel toward her. But the mother had not been staying overnight. Neither I nor the nurse I was working with that night had met her, so we harbored no ill-will.

That nurse proved marvelous. She was one of the two who had to repeat their orientation and was open about the fact that she wasn't the most talented of nurses. But she had a great knack for caring for people in a simple, honest way. About four a.m., Christy again quit breathing and her mother began crying out for us to "do something." Instead, the nurse held the mother and kept repeating, "Let her go, let her go." Despite the trying circumstances, Christy's dying had gone well. It almost certainly came on the very day she had chosen for herself—the day she turned fifteen.

Sadly, when the day-shift nurses arrived, both card-carrying members of the Stony Heart Brigade, I sensed no sympathy from them for the distraught mother or her daughter, just anger that we hadn't done the post-death preparations and hurried Christy's plastic-shrouded body off to the morgue. Looking back, I now realize that was a symptom of a problem eating at the heart of Hem-Onc. It would grow worse.

My nurse and I had a good reason for not doing the post-death procedures. We'd waited because the family had stayed in Christy's room with a Catholic priest until day shift arrived. It would have been totally out of place for us to force them out. The nurse I'd worked with that night could sense the anger from the day-shift nurses—an ill-tempered lot even in the best of times—but I told her not to worry. We'd done the right thing. On our shift, Christy had died properly. That's what mattered. Like it or not, day shift could handle the rest.

That experience with Christy also helped me to understand why Hippocrates, in his famous oath, focused on life's two extremes, calling for doctors to promise: "I will not give a lethal drug to anyone if I am asked, nor will I advise such a plan; and similarly I will not give a woman a pessary to cause an abortion."

At the beginning of our lives, we're vulnerable, unknown, and often friendless. Only an inviolate oath will protect us. At the end of life, we are equally vulnerable. Our departure creates no surprises and typically no investigation. If someone administers a poison to hasten death—and an excess dose of morphine is a poison—no one is likely to suspect. Both end-of-life situations then become entering wedges for the ever expanding use of death as treatment. You see that in Christy's case. When she stopped breathing, there was nothing to force me to ask her to breath again. I could have easily done nothing. I encouraged her to breathe, because that was the right thing for her and her family.

My Nights with Leukemia

Far more disturbing, if I had a nasty agenda, I could have smothered her using a pillow with no one being the wiser. In some countries that does happen, particularly with drugs as a means. And with each year that passes, there are still-greater financial incentives to speed up the deaths of vulnerable populations. That incentive doesn't just involve the soon-to-die—where little money is saved—it applies with even greater force to the troubled newborn, the disabled, the chronically sick, and the debilitated elderly. The real financially incentive to kill lies with those who will live on for months or even years. The longer they're likely to linger, the greater the savings from a speedy exit.

Of course, even at the extremes death doesn't always win. Sometimes a patient or family refuses to give up despite contrary medical advice. At this time, a friend was working as a nurse at a nearby university hospital's ICU. The cancer treatment for one of her patients had gone sour, and he had a lung infection that was raging out of control. Medically, he was a disaster area. His respirator, completely maxed out, was barely putting enough oxygen into his blood to keep him alive. His kidneys had shut down due to the chemotherapy, so he was getting dialysis. On top of that, he was in a deep coma with his EEG showing nothing but abnormal brain waves. It is hard to imagine someone in a worse condition still being alive or living much longer.

The hospital staff agreed that they should 'pull the plug' and let him die. But, as his nurse told me, "his family was from Southeastern Asia, and they never give up." The family told the hospital that, if it stopped treatment, they would take him home and care for him themselves. That was impossible, so a disbelieving hospital continued treatment.

Then one day a nurse, simply following procedure, took his hand and said, "If you can hear me, squeeze my hand." Amazingly, he squeezed. Shortly after that his kidneys began to function, his infection relented, and he came off the respirator. As my friend explained, only one month after he seemed at death's door, he was so healthy that he walked out of the hospital. He still had cancer but wasn't going to die anytime soon.

At my hospital, something similar happened. One of the more mysterious diseases for young children is the deadly Reye's Syndrome. The causes aren't well understood, but seem to be related to a recent viral infection and the use of aspirin. It begins with a headache and fever, but can progress to a deep coma, multiple organ failures, and death.

This boy had a case so severe that the hospital had no experience with anyone recovering, so the more aggressive treatment was stopped but—and here is the critical point—his IV was kept running to keep him hydrated. He was being *allowed* to die, but nothing was being done to *make* him die.

The nurse who told me his story was still amazed by what happened next. A nurse went into the boy's room to check on the IV, and he sat up and said, "I'm hungry." He soon recovered and went home.

Here, I've being talking about medicine at the extremes. I hope you understand that, at those extremes lie a variety of responses that call for thinking minds and warm hearts. With Pauline, the situation called for the hospital to get out of the way. It would have been cruel to decide that she ought to die in a hospital. She wanted to die at home, and that wish was honored.

Christy's situation was different. It called for gentle measures by me to restore her breathing so her family could arrive. At that point, it became right to simply 'let her go,' as her nurse said. And given her mother's inability to cope, Christy had to be in a hospital or hospice.

For that young man from Southeastern Asia, yet another response was right. His family, probably reflecting his own attitude, wanted to fight to the very end, and their resolve was respected. The absence of dictates from some governmental bureaucracy gave the hospital staff that freedom. That too was good. For all I know, he might still be alive.

Finally, for that little boy with Reye's Syndrome, the fact that halting what seemed to be futile treatment was not accompanied by schemes to hasten death—such as halting his IV—allowed him to live what is likely to be a long and healthy life. What medicine could not do, his own body did. It healed him. Medicine does not know everything and never will. Not everyone who seems fated to die, does die.

We should never forget the astonishing variety of situations that accompany dying or almost dying mean that the proper thing to do can never be written into rigid hospital protocols, least of all those generated by a far-away committee of self-styled experts. Different situations require applying, with intelligence and kindness, the differences that make us individuals. No distant bureaucracy—consulting only protocols, tables and statistics—can make those decisions. That's particularly true of a stony-hearted bureaucracy hypersensitive to costs.

26. FRIGHTENED JIMMY

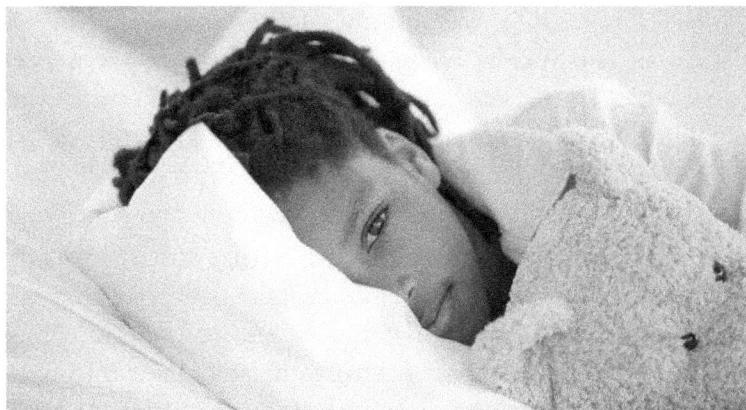

Normally, my relationship with the kids was an easy one. I brought them things they wanted, such as a blanket or a bowl of Jello, and I had a cute little Kola bear clipped to my stethoscope that they liked. Even more important, the medical stuff I did—typically taking vital signs every four hours—wasn't painful. They soon learned that someone in a short, white tunic like me wasn't going to hurt them. The people they feared were the medical technicians who wore long white coats and did blood draws. I'd go into the room and the kid would smile. A medical technician would go in a few minutes later and that same child would scream. It took real dedication for them to do that day after day.

Jimmy was an exception. He'd had such a bad experience with medicine that when he was first admitted he saw everyone as an enemy, even harmless me. I'd go into his room to check his blood pressure—high blood pressure was one of his problems—and he'd scream like I was torturing him. With his thin arms, taking his blood pressure was difficult enough. Screaming made it nearly impossible. Once, when a resident became upset at my difficulty getting accurate numbers, I challenged him to try. First, he made a go with his pricey stethoscope and drew a blank. Then he borrowed my ten-dollar one and still found the results dubious. I didn't have to tell him, "I told you so." I just did the best I could with this most unhappy little boy.

Jimmy had reason to be afraid. He was young black boy and, like Susie, the medical system had woefully failed him. When he was first admitted, his abdominal tumor was already huge. Anyone looking at his spindly arms and swollen belly could tell that something was badly wrong. A quick check would have discovered that sky-high blood pressure, and yet there'd been months of delay.

The one saving grace was Jimmy's father. He sometimes stayed nights and was able to calm his boy down. After a couple of weeks the boy smiled when I came into the room. The father told me of the difficulty the family had experienced in getting medicine to take Jimmy's condition seriously. One doctor, he said, wrote the boy's problems off as an eating or nutritional disorder, obviously without doing a close exam.

I had mixed feelings. On one hand, like that father, I was disgusted by the delay in Jimmy's treatment. There was no way that could be explained as anything other than incompetence or indifference. On the other hand, I wondered where that father had been during the delays. His presence, strong and articulate, was motivating the hospital to take his boy seriously. Had he been involved earlier on when the tumor might have been treatable? I couldn't imagine a doctor ignoring him. Sadly, medicine is like any other profession. Things often happen only because someone applies pressure. The boy's father certainly knew how to apply pressure, but had he been involved when it would have made a difference? That I don't know.

I thought of Jimmy a few years ago when I talked with a white South African who was founding an organization to deal with the many orphans that the AIDS epidemic has created in Africa. His solution was sensible and kind. AIDS in Africa is different, he told me. Most AIDS deaths involve young adults, both men and women. That not only left orphans behind, it meant grandmothers lost the support of their grown children. His orphanages were to be located in communities across Africa and would offer those grandmothers dignity and a place to stay while they cared for these orphans. In a sense, they would adopt those children as their own. It was a great idea.

He went on to tell me of a little twelve-year-old girl who was in similar situation to the Susie and Jimmy that I'd known. She had acquired AIDS, she knew not how, but her family wanted nothing to do with her, suspecting she had 'done something' to get it. He became almost her only friend, and she needed him. It was all too easy for South Africa's medical system to ignore a poor, dying little black girl all alone in the world, so he took her to medical appointments and stayed with her, using his power as a white, educated, well-connected adult man to make

My Nights with Leukemia

sure she got the best possible treatment. Nothing gets a hospital's attention like someone who can make trouble.

I knew what he meant. For a time I was the assistant director of a homeless shelter in Anchorage, Alaska. Our housing, in one giant dormitory room created from the auditorium of an old Pentecostal church, was for men only, while our meals were open to anyone.

One evening in late winter, a homeless woman showed up for a meal. She'd been living on the street for several weeks and had acquired a bad case of trench foot. The shelter's director told me to take her to the city's Native American hospital and do two things.

First, stay in the waiting room until a doctor came to treat her. Otherwise, he warned, they might ignore her, hoping she'd go away. From what she told me as we waited, that callousness had an excuse. She'd been in and out of that hospital so many times, she said, we'd know when her medical record arrived on the overhead conveyor. It'd be about two-inches thick.

Second, the shelter's director said, I was to leave as soon as a doctor came to examine her. If I didn't, he warned me, the hospital would try to put her care onto our shelter, which had no space for women, when what she needed was a lengthy stay in a warm, dry hospital bed. That's also what I did, and it worked.

In the end, much of Jimmy's treatment seemed driven more by professional guilt than genuine concern. His condition worsened, so he was transferred to the ICU. There, his cardiac arrest triggered a panic. A nurse who cleaned him up after he died told me that she had to remove over twenty IV needles from his frail little body. In his last few minutes, there'd been that many attempts to start an IV, attempts that they must have known were useless. Help came, but it came too late and with emotional baggage that was of no benefit to Jimmy.

Nor were cases of neglect or abandonment confined to impoverished minority children. In fact, the only time I saw a resident get angry with a child's parents came at the start of one night shift. A mother and father, white and in their late twenties, had brought in their son, who was about two. They insisted that he needed to be in the hospital. Examining the boy, the resident found a kid with nothing more serious than an ordinary case of the flu. There was no need for hospitalization, and a more senior physician would have bluntly told the parents that. But being new to the hospital, this resident lacked confidence, so the boy was admitted. Because he had an infection, he had to be placed in an isolation room.

As soon as he was admitted, his parents darted away. At that point, I became the angry one. This sick boy was being abandoned, pure and simple. He would spend the weekend in a room all by himself. There was no reason they couldn't have stayed. The isolation room had a fold-out bed they could have used.

Looking for justification, I checked the boy's chart. Maybe, I thought, they're from far away and have a long drive home. No, they were from a bedroom suburb a mere 20 minutes away. I also found the real reason this kid was being abandoned. They had a Medicaid coupon that covered the cost of this unnecessary hospitalization. Our hospital and the state were providing extremely expensive child care.

The boy was with us for three days. I went into his room whenever I could, but that wasn't nearly the attention he required. He needed his absent parents. When he got better, the hospital called them and told them to pick him up. As parents, they certainly weren't impressive. Nothing makes that more obvious than a sick child. When that boy got older, I suspect the roles reversed. The parents became the ones who were neglected.

My Nights with Leukemia

27. Families Matter

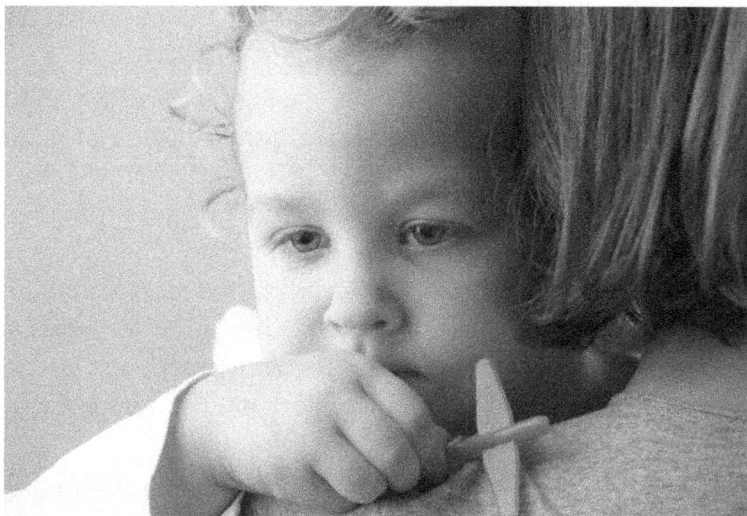

O ne social change worried me the most while I worked with these
sick children. That was the impact of our society's growing numbers of going-it-alone mothers. The mother of Eli, the first boy I cared
for who died, did support him to the very end, but the necessity of
working to pay bills meant she couldn't be with him at night. I filled
in for her as best I could, but I also asked myself what would have happened if my work load made it impossible for me to carve out 45 minutes each night to rock him to sleep.

And yes, little three-month-old Shana's single mom was able to stay
with her baby through the long days and nights. But that was only because the baby's father back in Saudi Arabia was willing and able to
provide financial support. Not all absentee fathers will and can do that.

It wasn't hard to see that these women's care for their children, as
heroic as it might be, was lessened by their circumstances. Two is almost always better than one. All alone, these stressed-out mothers had
a much more difficult time helping their child through an illness than
couples in a stable and close marriage. I saw that over and over again.
Having less themselves, they had less to give.

Adding to my worries about our future was a situation where a most
adorable boy with leukemia—I still have pictures of the smiling little
charmer—had a home situation so troubled, his grandmother had to

take over his care. She could do that because her own marriage was intact. She had a husband and didn't have to work to pay bills. "What's going to happen," I asked myself back then, "when both the parents and grandparents have broken homes and strained circumstances? Who is going to give these kids the emotional support they need?

It's crude, but there's an engineering analogy to having a child with cancer or some other severe illness. During their testing of a new aircraft, Boeing has one final test that they make on a wing to measure its breaking strength. They slowly bend that wing upward until it shatters. A sick or dying child puts a similar stress on a family, sometimes pushing it beyond the breaking point. The stronger, the more numerous, and the more intact a family is, the more likely it has the resources to give that child love and emotional support. The weaker it is, the less support a child gets. That can even lead to no support at all and tragedies such as the lonely deaths of Susie and Tanya.

Yes, I know. In some circles it's not politically correct to say what I'm saying here. Some would have us believe that women—totally unlike men—are superhuman beings only held back by out-dated stereotypes. That's nonsense. Working in Hem-Onc, the benefits of intact, two-parent families were all too obvious. At the most basic level, it usually meant the presence of a parent with the child almost all the time, particularly during those long and lonely nights. Sometimes it meant both parents stayed, especially if they were from out of town. At other times it meant that one of the pair, usually the mother, took on caring for their sick child, while the other, typically the father, concentrated on their other children and maintaining the family's income. Able to support one another, the parents had the emotional reserves to give their sick child love and attention. Like sailing a small boat in a storm, two is far more than twice one.

Also, even when a long and exhausting hospitalization meant that neither parent could manage to stay every night, the existence of a dad and a mom, united and able to cope, made a big difference for that child. With their home world safe and secure, the unfamiliar world of a hospital became less frightening. That was precisely the situation with Jackie, a girl I'll soon write about. Filling her nights with attention and love was far easier than filling a similar gap in Eli's life, much less that of Susie. Eli had only his mother, and Susie had no one. Jackie had both parents and two older brothers. She slept well.

Hospital staff, however much they might try, are only a partial solution for missing parents. With Eli, all I could offer him was help getting to sleep. I could do nothing about the terrors than haunted him nor could I be in the room if he woke up in the middle of the night. I had six other desperately sick kids to care for. That's why it was fortunate that, once asleep, he stayed asleep.

With Susie, I could not even give her a full night's sleep. She awoke over and over again. Only the loving care of a nurse, staying over on her own initiative, kept her from dying alone. For tiny and frail Tanya, a girl I'll write about later, only the presence of a fellow patient who bravely became her friend in her last weeks eased her dying.

In the case of Jackie, that meant that she needed me only as a nighttime friend, bottle feeder, and lullaby singer—practical things I could manage. The deeper emotional support she needed already came from her home. Again, the difference lay in their families—intact, two-parent families versus broken or never-formed families.

That brings up an issue that some may find touchy. It's a simple fact that two of the three worst cases of parental abandonment I saw were of black children. There was Susie, who was left to die all alone, and Jimmy, whose fatherly attention came too late and whose mother was never there. Only sad little Tanya, whom I will discuss later, had white parents. Why was that?

It certainly didn't reflect the ratio of the city's mostly white population nor, on close examination, did the lack of parents as they lay dying reflect the results of any racial bias on the hospital's part. Both Susie and Jimmy had conditions serious enough that, as soon as they were admitted, they were assigned private rooms in which someone in their family *could have* stayed each night. And once Tanya's situation grew more serious, she too had a private room. Yet two of the three never—as far as I knew—had a parent staying with them at night and none had a mother caring for them. Why was that?

I'll leave you to ponder that. Personally, I think it had little to do with race and much to do with the fact that black people simply happened to be a little further along the same disastrous, destructive path of single parenthood that so many whites are also troding.

Next, we'll examine events that are all too common in hospital—mistakes and blunders by physicians and staff.

28. Samantha's Misdiagnosis

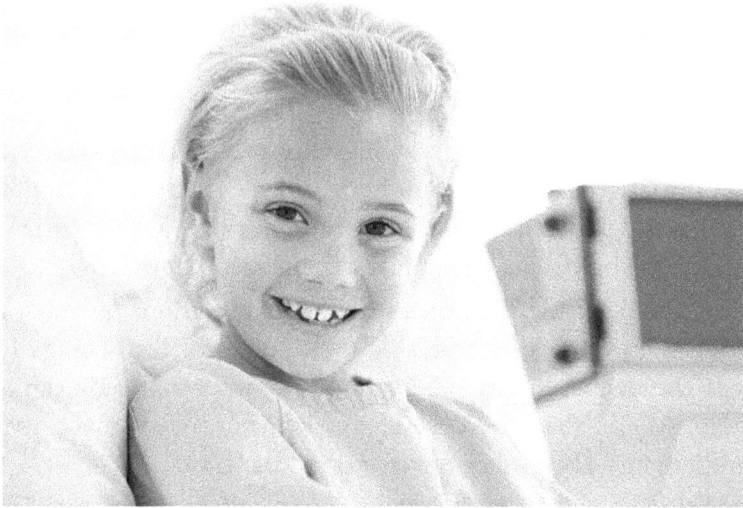

Her case was by far the most stomach-churning event that happened during my over two years at this hospital, and I suspect the nurses I was working with felt the same. In retrospect, this little girl's problem was so simple, only the tragedy of being assigned Dr. Most Stupid can explain what happened. I'm glad I didn't learn who he or she was, since I might not have behaved nicely. I suspect that doctor was as consumed by guilt as the rest of us were by anger and disgust.

Samantha was a five-year-old and so pretty her father dreamed of her becoming a model. He was with his much-loved daughter at a shopping center when she tried to pull away. Holding on to her arm, there was a snap, followed by a sharp pain in her left arm that didn't go away, leading to her admission. We were the top children's hospital in the region. Surely we would know what was wrong.

Later, I heard that what the little girl had was called 'shopping center arm.' I've not been able to find anything under that name today, but it's clearly an example of compartment syndrome. Medicine Online has this to say:

Compartment syndrome occurs when blood supply is dramatically reduced to muscles in a closed body space, known as a compartment. Compartments are found in the hand, forearm, upper arm, abdomen, buttock, and leg. The muscles most frequently involved are those on the front of the lower leg or the palm side of the forearm.

In Samantha's case, that meant the palm side her left forearm. There's also this remark in WebMD:

Compartment syndrome occurs when excessive pressure builds up inside an enclosed space in the body. Compartment syndrome usually results from bleeding or swelling after an injury. The dangerously high pressure in compartment syndrome impedes the flow of blood to and from the affected tissues. It can be an emergency, requiring surgery to prevent permanent injury.

A typical case involves a parent trying to restrain an over-eager child at a shopping center. The child tries to dart away and the parent hangs on to the child's arm, bringing the child to an abrupt halt. In a small number of cases, the resulting snap can cause a blood vessel to rupture in the child's arm, causing the sac-like fascia that surrounds the muscles to fill with blood. That brings pain. When the fascia fills completely, the supply of oxygen to muscles is cut off, leading to tissue death, with the pain often disappearing.

That's precisely what happened with lovely Samantha, but incredibly, that's not the diagnosis she received. In defiance of the evidence, Dr. Most Stupid concluded that she had an infection and prescribed antibiotics. Even worse, no one—myself included—pointed out the obvious: "Her skin wasn't broken. How could she get an infection?" Because it can look like other illnesses, compartment syndrome isn't easy to diagnose, but it should have at least been considered.

The first night, to my shame, I hardly noticed her. Children on IV antibiotics were so routine, those getting them were almost invisible. The second night, I did notice. She'd become unusual. If there was an infection, the antibiotic should have worked quickly. It hadn't, so compounding incompetence with utter folly, Dr. Most Stupid had ordered a warm wrapping for her arm to improve the circulation. Yes, slowly it was dawning on him (or her), that the problem might have something to do with circulation.

That's when Samantha's case belatedly drew my attention. Being a state-of-the-art hospital, we couldn't simply have a warm water bottle that I'd change every couple of hours. That'd have been too simple.

Nor could we have anything electrical in contact with a patient, like a heating pad that parents might use at home. That would have been considered too dangerous, particularly given the greed of the legal profession. Instead, when I came on duty we were using a machine the size of a window air-conditioner—I kid you not, it was huge—to circulate warm water through a pouch wrapped around her arm. At that point the thought passed through my mind, "This makes no sense. If we're having to do all this, she must not have an infection."

I still kick myself for not drawing attention to her that night. A few hours after I went home, the little girl's actual condition was discovered, Dr. Most Stupid's orders were shoved aside, and she was rushed into surgery. But by then, most of the muscles in her lower arm were dead and had to be removed. That's what made us so sick. For the rest of her life, her left arm would be thinner than her right. She'd have difficulty with any activity or sport that used her left arm.

That most horrible event completed a process that had begun with little Binky's too-rapid breathing because a nutritionist forgot he needed protein. After little Samantha, I made a solemn promise that I would no longer assume I was there simply to carry out orders. Those who were issuing the orders could make mistakes, terrible mistakes. As the staff member most in contact with our children, I might be their last and only hope. I needed to watch, to think, and to speak out.

Even more important, I now realized that some blunders triggered in me a sense of unease. Something deep inside me often knew when things were going wrong. When that feeling appeared again, I promised myself, I would pay attention and act.

But that raises a critical issue. How could a mere aide like me to get a physician's orders changed? Challenging orders wasn't in my job description. Following them was. Fortunately, I was beginning to know enough about how a hospital works to understand how to 'punch above my weight.' But I knew it wouldn't be easy.

First, I needed to do such good work that the hospital's pecking order mattered little. Being good at what I did would raise my statue. There is power in being right. People would get so used to trusting me, they'd listen when I said something that went against the flow.

Second, I could take advantage of the considerable power nurses had at my hospital. If a nurse chose to use that power, she had considerable authority. Win her to my side, and I would share her power.

What was that power? I was told about it during orientation. It was an established hospital policy that, if a nurse, even one fresh out of nursing school, objected to a treatment being given to a patient, a formal procedure must be followed. Day or night, the patient's attending physician had to be contacted, and the nurse permitted to make her case. If the attending refused to change the order, there was another step a nurse could insist on. The hospital's most senior physicians, the chiefs of medicine or surgery, would be called and forced to decide between her and the attending physician.

That's how Dr. Most Stupid's ridiculous order could have been changed. And yes, the whole process is strange, a bit like an enlisted soldier being permitted to challenge a general's orders. I was a private, and the nurse was a corporal. With her on my side, I could take on a misguided general. Just keep in mind that speaking up like that was risky. If the nurse and I were wrong, we might suffer consequences.

That said, there's nothing unusual about this policy. In numerous fields involving dangerous activities, certain people have the authority to invoke emergency rules that can't initially be questioned. A airplane pilot can declare an emergency and insist he be able to land quickly. If he does that, air traffic control must give him immediate clearance to any runway, even if dozens of other aircraft have to be scattered across the sky and air traffic disrupted for hours. Only later, if it's discovered that his emergency was bogus or ill thought out, can that pilot be disciplined. That's because in emergency situations, there's simply not enough time for a lengthy weighing process.

In a hospital, something similar is required to short circuit the normal process by which a nurse questions the wisdom of a doctor's orders. Normally, a night shift nurse might ask a day shift nurse to raise an issue when the physicians come around. In some cases that takes too long, hence those mandated, middle-of-the-night calls.

Third, as much as possible, I needed to put my objections into arguments that carry weight in a hospital. I couldn't talk about hunches and feelings. Medicine is more open to that today, but at the time, such a claim carried little weight. That meant I needed to understand the treatment we were giving, so I could to come up with arguments that fit how doctors think. Later, that would play a decisive role in two situations in which I had a gut-level feeling something was wrong.

Unfortunately, there was yet another disturbing fact that I made myself ponder. I might not always be able to persuade the nurse or resident on duty that night to my view. In the end, my commitment to making sure a bad order got rescinded could not depend on my ability to persuade anyone else. It had to take on the trapping of actual power. Even in the absence of a established hospital policy covering me, I had to find a way to force a change, come what may. I had to be able to shape events to my will. A child's life might depend on that.

Initially, I despaired at finding that only-up-to-me power. I was an aide, at least three steps down the pecking order from the physician who issued the orders. In a hospital, that's an immense gap. Eventually, I would discover an answer, but only during my final few weeks at the hospital. It was highly risky and invoking it might get me fired, but it would get a child much needed attention. I'll tell you about it later.

Before I close this chapter, I'll explain why I was beginning to consider myself knowledgeable enough to take on a system as awe-inspiring and intimidating as a top-tier hospital. It's actually simple. In some situations, hands-on experience matters more than formal expertise or book learning. Also, the attending physician, however capable, may not have seen a patient recently, and a patient's condition can change rapidly, particularly with children who have cancer.

The residents I was working with had only a few weeks experience on our unit. The night nurses, at that time often hired directly out of nursing school, typically had only a few months. By this point, my hands-on experience on Hem-Onc was several times that of any nurse I was working with. In fact, because I specialized on Hem-Onc, many nights I'd worked more hours there than all three of the unit's on-duty nurses combined and vastly more than the resident on duty that night. To deny that I could see a crisis developing was to deny that I'd learned anything in all those hundreds of hours.

Most important of all, I realized that in the end it would not depend completely on me. The senior physicians I wanted to wake up and draw into the decision typically had decades of experience. My experience may have trumped those I was working with, but their experience trumped mine. That expertise merely needed to be made aware of the changed circumstances.

Soon, I would need to call on my commitment to speak up whatever the cost.

My Nights with Leukemia

29. WENDY, SENSING DANGER

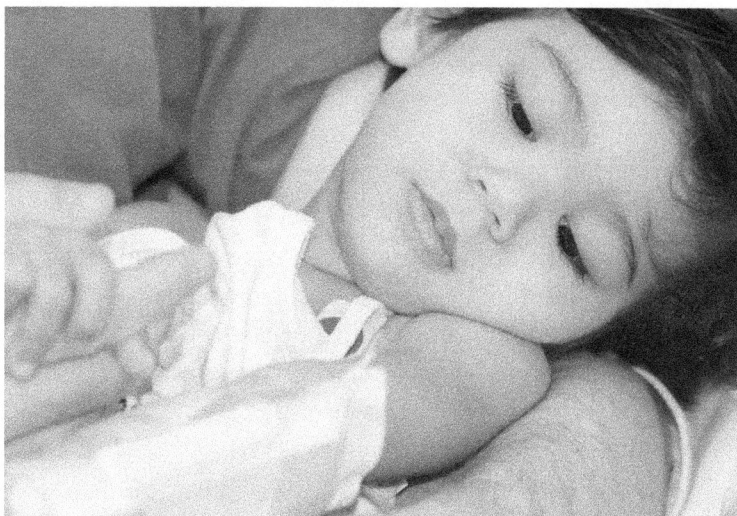

She'd be in before, and that's what made me uneasy. The last time we'd cared for hot-tempered, two-year-old Wendy, she'd scream whenever staff came near her. Only her mother could calm her. Now she seemed oblivious to everyone. She'd been grinding her teeth earlier in the evening, so we were using a homemade padded tongue depressor in her mouth. To give mom a break, I was holding her.

Wendy was a little more than 24 hours into what was supposed to be a 24-hour infusion of chemotherapy for her leukemia. Interruptions had added enough delay that it'd take an extra two hours to finish. That happened often and wasn't normally an issue. The resident had just approved the extension and left to catch a few hours sleep in his miserable 32-hour shift. Her mother had gone for coffee, and the nurse had returned to her other duties, leaving me with this out-of-it little girl.

I sat there, growing increasingly troubled. Wendy wasn't just acting differently from her last visit. She was acting odd by any measure. She didn't seem to know her mother had left or that I was holding her. In fact, she didn't seem aware of anything. Sometimes we drugged into oblivion kids who didn't want to deal with the nausea that chemotherapy could trigger. But she hadn't been drugged. She was simply acting like no kid in her situation should act. I decided to take a momentous first step. I'd challenge that just-issued medical order and by implication the one issued earlier by the attending physician. "Something is wrong," I told myself. "This chemotherapy must stop."

Wendy was in my lap, so I stood up enough to reach the call light. Since the nurse would know it was me calling for her, she'd come quickly. I sat down to figure out how to transform my gut-level intuition into something medical—something with numbers or at least with the proper indications. Get my nurse with me and perhaps she could persuade the resident to stop the treatment. Smart residents listened to nurses, but I wasn't that sure about the one that night. He had his quirks.

Fortunately, I didn't need an argument. A few seconds after I hit the call light, Wendy's left foot began to twitch. I've seen enough seizures to know what was happening. Before this one struck, I had her in the bed on her side and was gently restraining her, so she wouldn't hurt herself. When the nurse arrived about thirty seconds later, I no longer needed to give a reason to stop the chemotherapy.

Yes, my nurse may have thought I'd hit that call light *after* the seizure began, and I didn't see any reason to tell her otherwise. But what mattered was that the seizure said it all. I needed no other argument. This little girl was in serious trouble. The resident was called, and the chemotherapy stopped. After the attending physicians arrived the next morning, Wendy was transferred to the ICU. I never found out what had gone wrong, but since she also had an Ommaya reservoir draining her spinal fluid, I assume it was some complication related to that.

At this point, I knew my attitude had changed from passive to active. I'd acted differently with Wendy, because I had learned something from my too-silent blunders with Binky's rapid breathing and with Samantha's wrapped arm. I now listened to my experience-honed instincts.

Years later, what I was grasping at—an intuitive sense that something is wrong that later proves true—was described by Gary Klein in his ground-breaking 1998 book, *Sources of Power: How People Make Decisions*. His studies form the basis for much of Malcolm Gladwell's best-selling *Blink: The Power of Thinking Without Thinking* (2005). It seems that I wasn't alone in learning to 'trust my gut.' Experienced professionals have always done precisely that.

In the fourth chapter of his book, Klien explains his research into how firefighters make decisions in situations where seconds count and lives hang in the balance. In one, a lieutenant described an apparently simple fire in the kitchen of a modest home. He and his men entered and pumped water on the fire. "Odd," he thinks, "The water should have had more of an impact." They try again, but the fire roars back. Something, the lieutenant realizes, isn't right. He orders his men to leave the building. Moments later, the floor where they'd been standing collapsed. This home may have looked like all the other one-story homes in the neighborhood, but it was different. It had a basement and the fire was there rather than in the kitchen. That's why the fire had come back despite their efforts.

Nurses have similar experiences. Later in that same chapter Klein describes research that one of his co-workers, Beth Crandall, did for the National Institute of Health. One of the most difficult decisions Neonatal Intensive Care Unit (NICU) nurses have to make is deciding when one of their tiny babies has an infection. For older children and adults there's usually enough time after clear signs of an infection develop for antibiotics to work. With these tiny babies, there often isn't. By the time an infection is detected and treatment began, it may be too late.

The most mysterious thing, Crandall discovered, was that some nurses—generally the more experienced ones—could tell physicians when their little patients were developing an infection, often a day or more in advance of any lab test. When asked, they said that they didn't know how they knew, that they simply knew. That's what Gladwell means by "thinking without thinking." We can know reliable truth without engaging in a conscious, rational, step-by-step process. That truth simply appears in our minds fully formed and demanding action.

Beth Crandall questioned these ICU nurses intensively, focusing on specific incidents. Some of the cues, she discovered, "were the same as those in the medical literature, but almost half were new, and some cues were the *opposite* of sepsis [infection] cues in adults. For instance, adults with infections tend to become more irritable. Premature babies, however, become less irritable. If a microbaby cried every time it was lifted to be weighed and then one day it did not cry, that would be a danger signal to the experienced nurse. Moreover, the nurses were not relying on any single cue. They often reacted to a pattern of cues, each one subtle, that together signaled an infant in distress."

There was to be another situation in which I would find myself following cues. This time I wouldn't need a fortuitous seizure. I would come up with a medical argument—poor as it was—and get action just in time.

30. Oblivious Brian

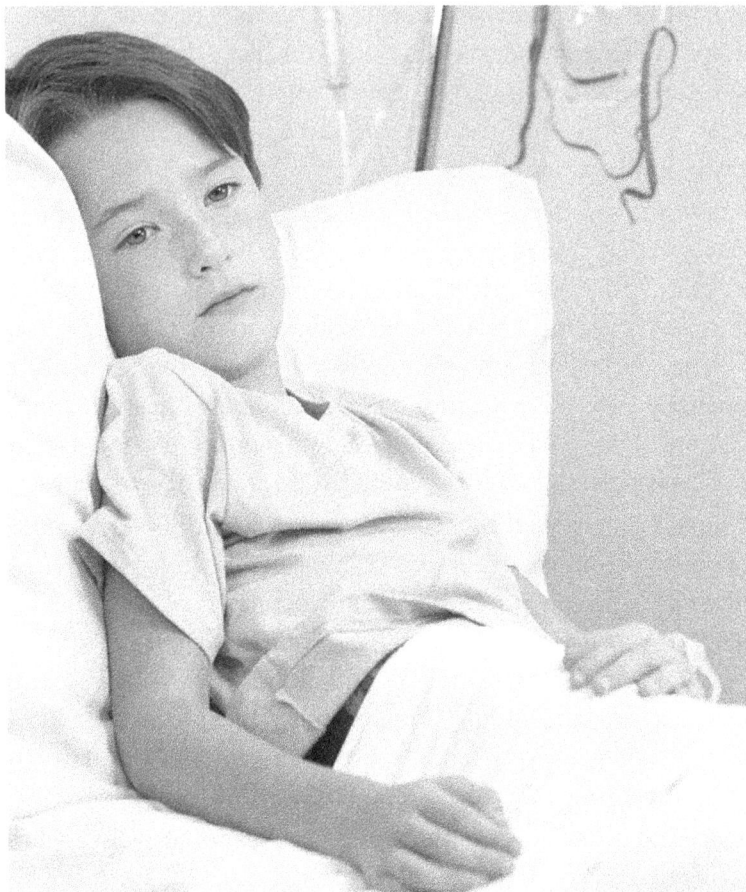

Brian illustrates just how quickly we moved with our leukemia patients. When I'd left the hospital on Friday morning, he wasn't a patient and quite possibly hadn't even been diagnosed. As I came on duty late Sunday evening, he'd been diagnosed and classified. Treatment orders had been written, and he was finishing his 24-hour induction chemotherapy. That's how fast we often acted, even on weekends.

About 1 a.m. that Monday morning Brian had a nosebleed that wouldn't go away, causing him to vomit. Messy stuff tended to be my job, so I was with him, holding a small bucket. About an hour later, the usual remedies for a nosebleed—sitting up, a compress, and then a cold compress—hadn't worked, so the resident took one final step. He began stuffing cotton wadding up that nine-year-old boy's nose. It was a brutal procedure made all the worse by the fact that I hadn't seen any local anesthetic given.

That's when the nagging thoughts began—the 'thinking without thinking.' "How can Brian take this so passively?," I asked myself. The stuffing had to be painful, and yet he was lying there, as oblivious to all that was happening as Wendy had been to her surroundings a few months earlier. I also knew he hadn't been like that an hour earlier when he'd been vomiting. Then, he'd been alert enough to be miserable.

I didn't blame the resident for how painful the nose stuffing was. Our doctors-in-training were still learning, so we had to cut them some slack. When he finished clumsily stuffing the boy's nose, the bleeding did stop. Were Brian's troubles over? I couldn't shake the feeling they weren't—that his nosebleed might mean more than low platelets and that his obliviousness meant something far worse.

That's when I tried to think medically. The boy had been admitted with a platelet count that was low—around 50,000. That might explain his nose bleed but not the rest. I knew the resident had just written up an order for a CBC (Complete Blood Count) to monitor those platelets. In a few seconds he would be returning to a room filled with bunk beds where tired residents caught naps in the middle of the night. If I were going to act, I had to move quickly.

On little more than a hunch, I went up to resident and suggested that he also order a blood chemistry test. The boy had been vomiting, I pointed out, so his electrolytes might be out of balance. He took my advice and wrote out an order.

I knew what I'd told him was poor. Brian hadn't done that much vomiting. But I also knew that something was wrong with Brian that merited more examination, and that test was all I had to go with. There was method to my madness. Because leukemia is a blood cancer, two common tests—a complete blood count and a blood chemistry—give a good overview of a patient's status. Something told me that'd be enough. I was 'thinking without thinking.'

The test proved enough. That resident should have thanked me, because I'd saved his neck. Just after I left work that morning, the results of that blood chemistry test came back with all alarms ringing. Brian's electrolytes were so out of whack, he was rushed to the ICU. When I came on duty that evening, he was back on the floor, already getting—

early and in high doses—the antidote that we normally gave to counter the chemotherapy after a 24-hour delay. Thanks to the test I'd gotten ordered early, he was recovering quickly.

The story doesn't end there. All that happened in the wee hours of Monday morning. Three nights later on Thursday, the evening nurse gave us the emerging picture. From the start, Brian had been an unusual patient. The 'acute' in his leukemia was particularly so, with extremely high numbers of evil 'blasts' circulating in his blood. That was one reason for the rush to treat. But those cancerous cells, the doctors now knew, were exceptionally sensitive to chemotherapy. Long-term, that was good news. His cancer was beatable. Short-term it meant trouble. Our chemotherapy triggered a massive cellular die-off. The cells breaking up and dumping their contents into his blood sent his electrolytes dangerously out of balance. Undiscovered, that might have killed him.

Today, Brian's problem is known as tumor lysis syndrome or TLS, which Medscape notes, "refers to the constellation of metabolic disturbances that may be seen after initiation of cancer treatment. It usually occurs in patients with bulky, rapidly proliferating, treatment-responsive tumors." My hunch was right in every way. A blood chemistry test is how it's diagnosed.

As a result of what happened to Brian, the evening nurse went on, the nation's top leukemia specialists had conferred and agree to change the national protocol governing the treatment of all children with leukemia. In the future, for cases like Brian's they'd no longer hit the ground running. Chemotherapy would start more cautiously, testing its effects.

"That," I thought, "is impressive. These doctors really do care. On Monday, they discover a problem with their current treatment. By Thursday, they've come up with a way to make sure it doesn't happen again." If only our society's other problems could be dealt with that fast and that definitively.

I also felt good inside. "Yes," I told myself, "all you did was speed up the process. When Brian didn't wake up Monday morning, there'd have been a 'stat' [instant] order for blood tests, and the problem would have been discovered in minutes." My quiet intervention merely sped up that discovery by an hour or two. Still, what happened that night did indicate that I was learning to bend the system in the right way. Even if no one had noticed, I'd made a difference. That felt good.

My Nights with Leukemia

31. A Warning about Jackie

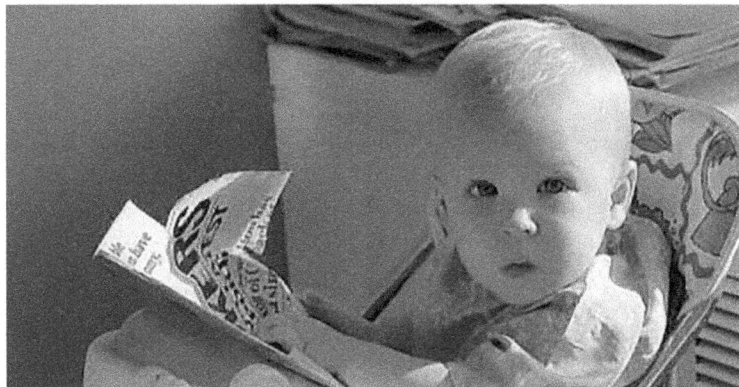

When I saw that black box with bold lettering in the Physician's Desk Reference (PDR, I knew all too well what it meant. It's the strongest warning the FDA can give about a drug's ill effects. The mysterious drug was for treating viral infections and to be used only for severe, life-threatening emergencies. You only gave it to a patient who'd die without it. The warning included a long list of scary side effects. That explained my orders to monitor most carefully this baby girl—the very one whose pictures you'll see at the start of each of her chapters.

Jackie, the baby girl who was getting this most wicked drug, had a rough time from the start. I remembered when she first arrived on our unit some six weeks earlier, diagnosed with a leukemia so rare, we were told there were only 32 cases in all medical literature. At six months, she was the youngest ever reported.

She wasn't my patient when she first arrived. When I came back after two days off, she'd already been admitted, developed problems, and gone into the quasi-ICU status we used in special cases. She was still on Hem-Onc, but had a nurse assigned to her around the clock. A special duty nurse meant no need for an aide.

Keep in mind that at that point we had not begun to treat Jackie's leukemia. Her troubles came from elsewhere. Keeping a traditional IV going on a small child is difficult and often means a new poke every two or three days, adding still more misery to an already terrible sickness. That's why putting in a central line was often our first step in treating leukemia. The line was a flexible Silastic (rubbery) tube that entered the upper chest and went into a large vein just before it returned to the heart. It could stay in place for months and also be used for blood draws, sparing a child still more pokes. We loved those lines, we were skilled in using them, and ordinarily there were no complications.

But with little Jackie, matters were always more complicated. The central line they'd surgically installed developed bleeding and a serious infection. A day later, she left us for the ICU. There she spent six long weeks, with doctors telling her family that her chances of leaving the ICU alive were less than two percent.

She beat back the challenge. When she returned to us, I found a lead-filled bag in her crib. It had pressed on her chest to stem the bleeding. I remember hefting it and thinking, "I'd hate to sleep with this on my chest. It must have been miserable for a baby." Jackie's will to live, an ICU nurse later told me, kept them treating her despite the terrible odds. She was one strong-willed little girl.

Her bleeding halted but still battling that viral infection, Jackie had returned to us, but she still required special attention. That was why she was getting the drug and the close monitoring it required. That's why I'd looked up her mystery drug.

It was then that something unique happened. If you work with exceptionally sick children, it's normal to feel sympathy for them and perhaps to develop a special liking for some. Liking was usually all that was needed. All our Hem-Onc patients had private rooms with a hideaway bed for their parents and, for almost all of them, at least one parent stayed through the night. As staff, we merely needed to do our job as kindly as possible. Their parents handled the child's emotional needs.

But Jackie's parents were exhausted by those long weeks in the ICU and had other children who needed their attention. They had learned to trust the staff, so they weren't staying overnight. Jackie was all alone, and incredibly hungry. Even though she was now eight months old, battling for her life had left her too weak to hold a bottle. If she was going to be fed, I'd have to hold it for her.

Much is born of necessity. To do what I could for Jackie, I became more disciplined than ever. All the care I gave other children had to be carefully managed to do the near impossible—free up an hour in the middle of the night to feed and give attention to this little girl who wanted so much to live.

32. Jackie and Three Beeps

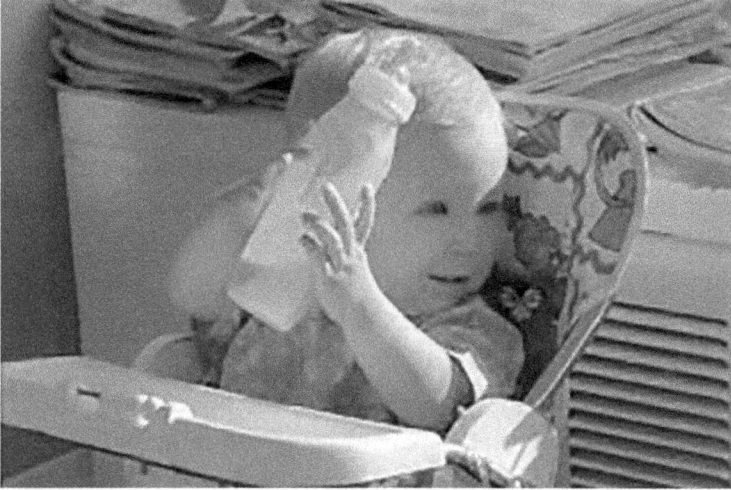

It was the middle of the night. I'd just finished my four a.m. vital signs and the nurse her four a.m. medications. She'd left on break, and I'd settled down for Jackie's bottle feeding. She was in my lap, and I'd just placed the bottle in her mouth when it happened. One of the IV pumps on Hem-Onc began to beep. With the nurse gone, I went to take care of it, after putting an unhappy Jackie back in her crib.

Returning, Jackie and I settled down again. Then another IV pump beeped, and I had to leave her yet again. This time she cried because, as you can see from the photo at the start of this chapter, she loved that bottle. I hurried back as fast as possible, but it was clear that she was now upset. Settling down once again, I'd just given her the bottle for a third time when another IV pump beeped. By this point, I was getting ticked off myself and wondering what was going on. Would those beeps never stop?

What was going on should have been obvious from the start. The nurse had ran her 4 a.m. medications and started the usual follow-up 15 cc rinses to clear medicine out of the line. Then she'd left on break, depending on me to convert the IVs from medication-dispensing to a maintenance drip. That happened all the time and was so normal, she'd not even reminded me. Those beeps coming some two minutes apart had been the result of her making her rounds and starting rinses.

Now knowing what was happening, I made sure there'd be no more beeps by checking the status of every IV pump on Hem-Onc. Then I went back to a most unhappy little Jackie. She took the bottle, of course, but was so ticked off that I'd betrayed her—me of all people—that she wouldn't even look at me for the rest of that night. "That's OK," I thought, "you know I care about you."

Later she got even, I like to pretend, for that thrice-fold abandonment. Several nights later, I'd just settled down with her and that bottle, when she had an "Oh that felt good" expression. In an instant, I thought, "Oh no, I forgot the rubber pad!" Here's a detail you may find useful if you're ever in a hospital with a baby to hold. Cheap disposable diapers of the kind hospitals buy leak badly, so always keep a rubber pad in your lap. A warm, wet feeling confirmed that.

In the end, all was fine. I continued to feed her. Afterward, I headed for the teen unit, borrowed a pair of jeans the right size and changed into them. Then I washed and dried my regulation white pants in Rehab's laundry, changing back to the proper attire before day shift arrived. On night shift you learn to make do with what you have.

Keep in mind the larger story behind these two amusing interludes, as well as why I describe them here. Jackie had been diagnosed with an extremely rare form of leukemia, one so rare, particularly in someone so young, that our physicians had no idea what her treatment should be. They were going on a guess, giving her the standard treatment for more ordinary forms of leukemia. We were in uncharted territory, so no one knew her chances of living or dying.

I was also finding myself in uncharted emotional territory. All too often books, movies and television give us distorted views about what life is like at the extremes. Earlier, I pointed out that mountain climbing could include both beauty and death at the same time. The same is true of medicine. The serious and sublime can blend with the silly and even funny—nasty anti-viral drugs with leaky diapers. Working with children battling cancer also brought joys and miseries mixed in unique ways. It's a poor writer or creator of a documentary who would portray work in Hem-Onc as unrelieved doom and gloom—or of sentimental sweetness and light like a sentimental Victorian novel. The two feelings mixed in ways that are difficult to put into words. The Book of Common Prayer says it best in the funeral service when it notes with great eloquence that, "In the midst of life we are in death." Life in the midst of death was what Hem-Onc was all about.

Friendships are often born of happenstance and necessity. That's how Jackie and I came together. In her desperate situation, she needed me, and I found myself there to help. It wasn't a conscious choice. It simply happened. Life is like that.

Now for a treat. Here's a picture of her having fun that morning ripping the the pages out of old magazines.

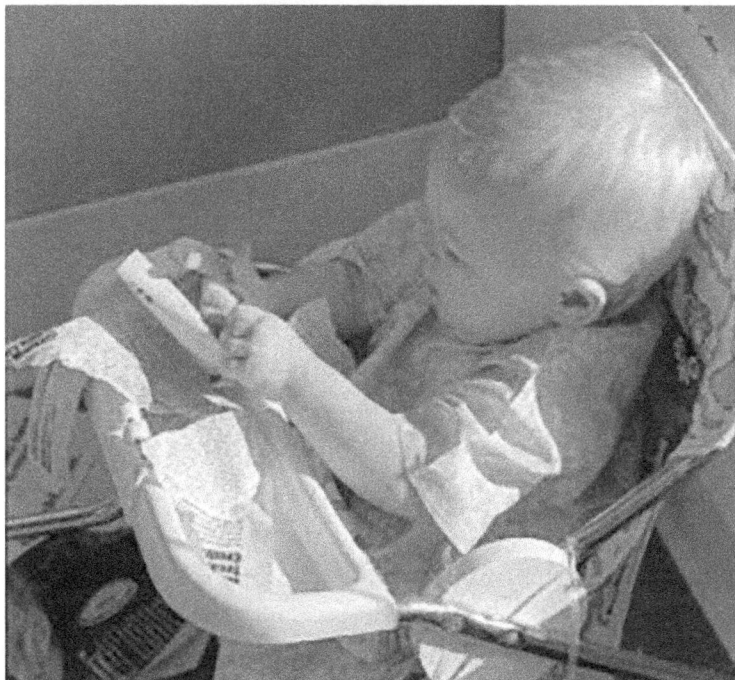

33. WHAT IF JACKIE DIES?

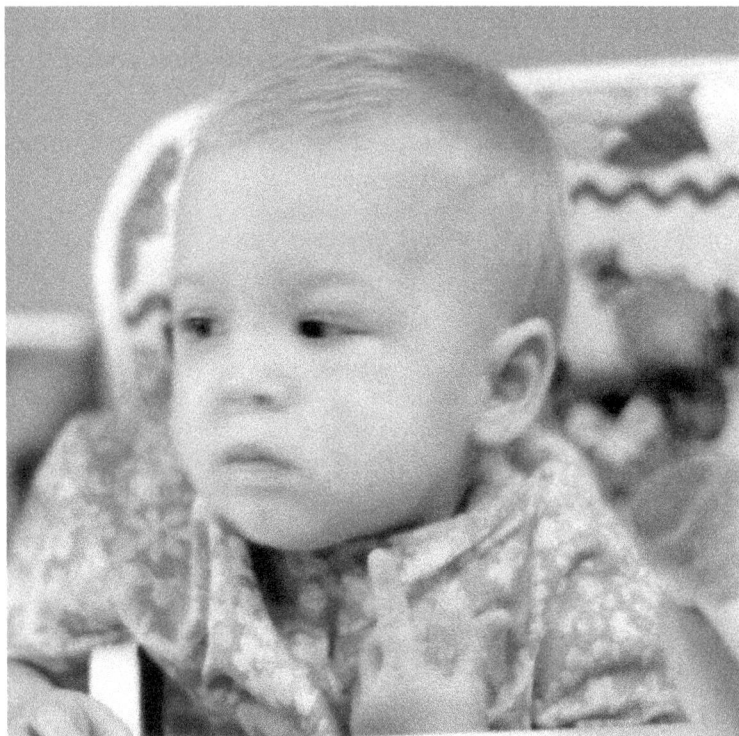

The nurse's question was blunt. "What will you do if Jackie dies," she asked me. I didn't know what to say, so I stood there mute and awkward. She asked again, and I still had no answer. The deaths of other kids had been like riding a train through a dark tunnel. I would miss them, but even at the darkest point, I knew the light would return.

Jackie's death, I sensed, would not be like that. I wasn't sure what would happen, but I knew it'd be more like a head-on collision with an oncoming train. In modern physics what I was facing is called a singularity—a situation so unique and overwhelming, its outcome cannot be predicted by anything in our experience. For me, Jackie's death would be unique. She wasn't just another patient. She was much more than that. I didn't know how I'd respond or what I'd be like afterward. For the first and only time, I was experiencing a little of what these children's parents must face each and every day.

The nurse wasn't being cruel. She was trying to help. She knew me and was making sure I understood what I faced. Behind her questioning lay the deeper questions that haunted almost everyone who worked on Hem-Onc, "What will happen if I fall for one of these kids? Is that something I should take care to avoid? Should I feign concern, so I don't look cold and uncaring, but keep my actual feelings aloft and distant?" From the start, my answer to the latter had been no. I'd decided that I wouldn't do that. I'd trust God and let the consequences fall where they may. Now I must live with that decision.

You get a fleeting glimpse into all that Jackie had gone through in the picture that opens this chapter, one taken the same times as the others. Notice the tired and almost haunted look that appeared in her eyes when she wasn't distracted by me, a bottle, or the sheer fun of tearing magazines apart. That's hints at how difficult her short life had been. She'd be through much in the preceding few months.

Remember too that these pictures were taken weeks after she'd come to us from the ICU, too weak to even hold a bottle. Her returning hair shows that she's in remission and almost recovered from her chemotherapy. And no, I never understood where that oft-repeated hand gesture she's making came from. Perhaps that's how she wrapped her fingers around the wires that monitored her in the ICU.

Through those dark nights with Jackie, I often reminded myself of what C. S. Lewis wrote in his great classic, *The Four Loves*. Near the end, he deals with the perils of love, referring to what St. Augustine wrote after the death of a friend. "This is what comes, he [Augustine] says, of giving one's heart to anything but God. All human beings pass away. Do not let your happiness depend on something you may lose."

Lewis concedes that a part of him finds that appealing: "Of all the arguments against love none makes so strong an appeal to my nature as, 'Careful! This might lead you to suffering.'" But he goes on to write: "When I respond to that appeal I seem to myself to be a thousand miles away from Christ. If I am sure of anything I am sure that His teaching was never meant to confirm my congenital preference for safe investments and limited liabilities." Then come the words I recalled often during the nights when Jackie's life hung by a thread.

There is no escape along the lines St. Augustine suggests. Nor along any other lines. There is no safe investment. To love at all is to be vulnerable. Love anything, and your heart will certainly be wrung and possibly be broken. If you want to make sure of keeping it intact, you must give your heart to no one, not even to an animal. Wrap it carefully round with hobbies and little luxuries; avoid all entanglements; lock it up safe in the casket or coffin of your selfishness. But in that casket—safe, dark, motionless, airless—it will change. It will not be broken; it will become unbreakable, impenetrable, irredeemable. The alternative to tragedy, or at least to the risk of tragedy, is damnation. The only place outside of Heaven where you can be perfectly safe from all the dangers and perturbations of love is Hell.

The nurse who was questioning me that night was persistent. She changed her question to another. "Why did I like Jackie?" she asked. I thought a moment and decided that was easy to answer: "Because she and I are alike." "How were we alike?," she wanted to know. In a flash I saw the answer, "Because we're both stubborn."

And stubborn we were. About a decade ago I faced a copyright legal dispute where the opposing party, one of the wealthiest literary estates on the planet, thought that I'd take the easy way out and give in. "Don't you realize" I felt like telling those nasty Manhattan lawyers, "that I will fight you to the bitter end, and I *will* find a way to win?" I've often thought of writing a book about that experience and calling it *Lawyers Are from Mordor.* Some lawyers are like that.

I won that dispute, making such a good argument for fair use for *Untangling Tolkien*, my day-by-day chronology of *The Lord of the Rings*, that the judge dismissed their lawsuit "with prejudice." That's a judge's way of saying to them, "Drop this lawsuit. You have no chance of winning."

Of course stubbornness like Jackie's and mine has a downside. During my first quarter in college, I took a survival swimming class where my stubbornness was all too obvious. And while it was certainly not death-defying—the coach and other students would not have let me drown—it did have me thumbing my nose at danger.

It happened this way. At the end of every class, we dove in two at a time and were expected to swim the length of the pool and back underwater, roughly 20 yards each way or 120 feet (40 meters) total. My lungs and heart are strong, so on the first day of class, I was one of the few who made it. As the quarter continued, more people did.

On the last day of class, we faced a brutal final exam to test what we'd learned. Without a moment's break, we had to demonstrate all the water survival techniques we'd been taught. After some fifty minutes in the water, we were exhausted and out of breath. With no chance to rest, we lined up for our final there-and-back underwater swim. I was already an hour late for a makeup chemistry lab, so I went first, paired with the classes' best swimmer, a former lifeguard. As soon as I hit the water, I was out of breath.

At that point, my motive was vanity. Today, I thought, it'll be impossible for anyone to cover that distance underwater. I'll swim as far as my partner, and there'll be no shame in that. He was a far better swimmer, so he pulled well ahead of me, turned around in the murky water, and started back. Drawn on by him, I kept swimming, even though my lungs were about to burst.

About half-way back, it was no longer about appearances. I now believed I could make it if I simply refused to give up. The last thing I remember were the grates at the deepest part of the pool, some ten feet from the end. Then everything went black. The next thing I knew, I was gasping for air as I was being yanked out of the water by my classmates. I'd made it—just barely.

I stumbled off to the showers to wash and shake off an urge to vomit. A short time later, the lifeguard came into the shower, a big smile on his face. He'd stayed to watch all those who'd made the swim successfully on the first day. "You're the only one to make it every time," he said.

"Didn't you make it?," I asked. That's what I thought I'd seen. "No," he answered, "I came up for air at the far end." At that time I was too sick to say anything. Later it came to me that I should have thanked him for keeping me going—for drawing me along behind him. He— along with my inate stubbornness—had let me to do the seemingly impossible.

That's how I was helping Jackie during those long nights. By being a part of her struggle and demonstrating that I cared for her and believed she could make it, I was drawing her along, helping her fight for life. My stubborn refusal to give up was buttressing her own stubbornness.

Equally important, I was doing everything in my power to give her the best possible chance at life. I watched her like a hawk. When she needed to be fed, I would find the time. If she as much as burped, I asked myself what that meant. Together we would make it.

34. You Are my Sunshine

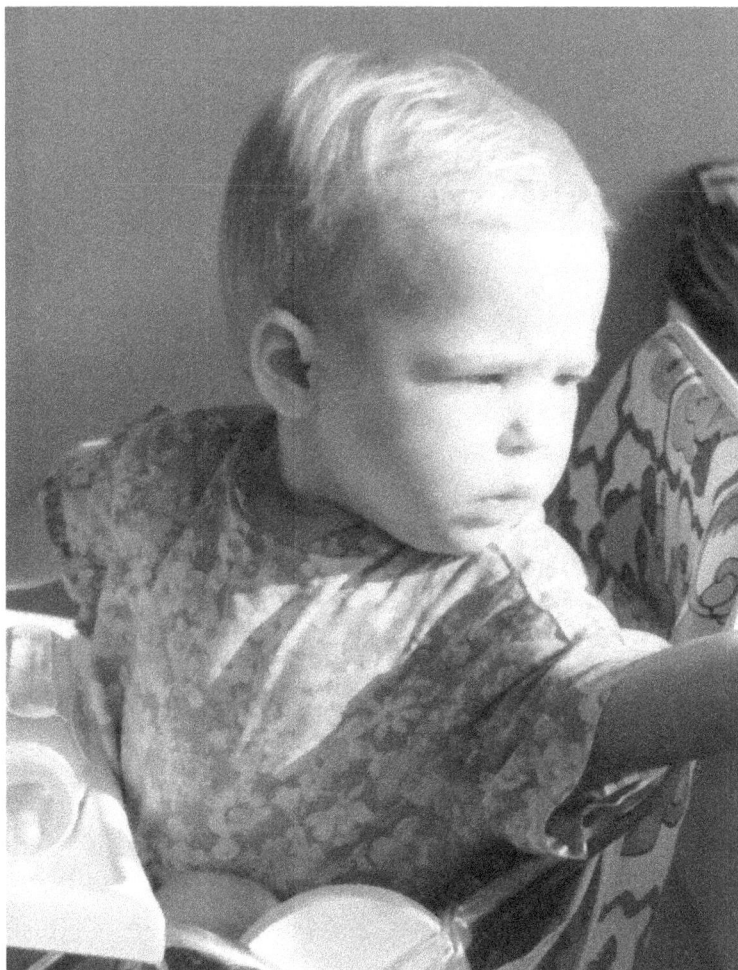

I don't know when I first heard the song. It must have been as a small child, because, when I would sing it to Jackie during bottle time, I thought it was a kid's lullaby. She certainly seemed to regard it as such, looking at me with wide-open eyes. Alas, I'm such a terrible singer, only small children appreciate my voice. Everyone else notices my flat monotone and cringes.

Since then I've learned that "You Are My Sunshine" is actually a romantic country and western song dating back to the late 1930s, and that its beautiful melody is almost identical to a traditional Ukrainian folk song. Go to YouTube and you'll find dozens of adaptations, some by the biggest names in popular music and others by amateurs accompanied by red valentines and cute kittens. The music and lyrics, simple as they are, strike deep cords in the human heart. Songs like it are so calming for babies and small children, learning them should be required in medical and nursing schools.

At the time I thought I was simply keeping little Jackie entertained with a silly lullaby. Only later did I realize that the words of the only part I knew, the chorus, held a special meaning for the two of us. While I was singing to her, I was also singing to myself. Here are the lines and what they must have meant.

You are my sunshine, my only sunshine.

Remember what I said about beauty existing alongside danger in mountain climbing and joy alongside tragedy in a hospital? This is the joy, illustrated by sunshine. That's what Jackie and I experienced that morning when she and I went to the play area and ripped magazines to shreds as a bright early morning sun poured in the windows. Fortunately, I had my camera with me that day, so I captured the pictures you've been seeing.

You make me happy when skies are grey.

Those nights in the hospital were certainly grim enough that more that a little happiness was desperately needed. It was a time for heeding Jesus' words about not borrowing worries and cares from tomorrow. Today has enough troubles. Let the sunshine carry you through the grey.

You'll never know dear how much I love you

Here the musical plot gets more complicated. I knew that I wasn't part of Jackie's family, that I was one of the hospital staff, placed there to care for her for a short time. I also knew that, when babies grow into children, they forget most of what happened to them when they were young, including the people who pass through their lives. Other than perhaps retaining a vague affection for someone who looks like me, I doubted she'd remember me, hence the "you'll never know."

Please don't take my sunshine away

Yes, that's where the song's message becomes so obvious, I can't explain why I was so clueless, much less why I persisted in thinking I was singing an innocent little lullaby. "Don't die," I was telling her over and over again during those nights. "I'll miss you terribly if you do."

In the end, my musical prayers were answered. Months later and safely in remission, her mother found me, now working days with teens, and brought my little sunshine along. Jackie had grown so much, I hardly recognized her, but she knew me and flew out of her mom's arms in her delight at seeing me and wanting to be held.

Jackie and I met one last time. A couple of months later, I was grabbing a quick lunch in the crowded hospital cafeteria, when I heard a 'ting' as a piece of silverware hit the floor nearby. I thought nothing of it until a few seconds later, when I heard another 'ting.' I turned around, and there was clever little Jackie looking at me from a high chair with a mischievous smile on her face. Speaking was still a bit much for her, so she'd hit on dropping silverware to get my attention. It worked.

That brief reunion proved to be the last time I saw her. I left the hospital soon afterward and turnover at the hospital was so high that within a couple of years I'd lost touch with almost anyone who could bring me news. Several years later, however, I ran into one of the volunteers at the Ronald MacDonald house. Knowing of my interest in Jackie, he told me that she'd just passed a major milestone—five years without a relapse. That was good news, very good news indeed. My little sunshine was still shining.

Now we must turn to matters far less sunny. That's the often unpleasant world of hospital politics. Get ready. We're entering darker and more depressing times. Prepare yourself.

35. Sicker Kids?

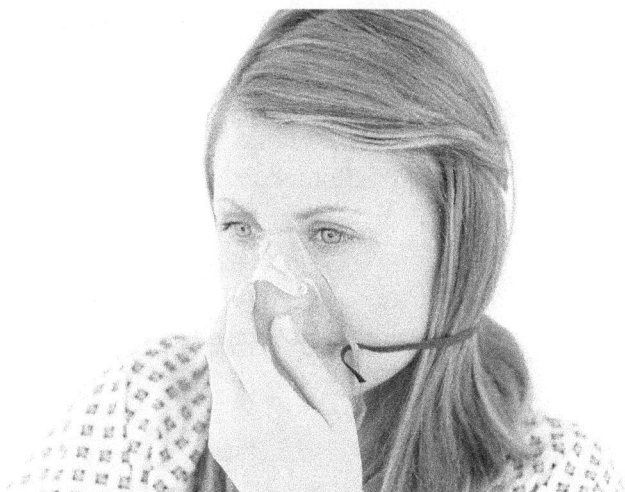

Her words would prove prophetic. "About every five years," this experienced nurse was telling me, "this hospital goes off on a tangent." The last time it happened, she went on to explain, was several years before when doctors in the community became convinced that having a patient admitted meant they lost all contact with the child and his parents. The hospital was saying, in effect, "Get lost. You've done all you can. We're the experts. You're not needed anymore."

The doctors in the community were most unhappy. Once discharged, the child would become their responsibility again. They needed to know what had happened. The result, she said, was a disaster. Doctors found other hospitals for their patients. So few beds were occupied, she went on, that entire units had to be shut down. Financially, it was a dark time for the hospital and those who worked there.

I didn't doubt her. What she described wasn't a problem someone would invent. Later, what she told me was confirmed when I found, at the back of a nursing station drawer, a pin whose exact wording I don't recall, but whose meaning was obvious. It called on the hospital's staff to treat physicians out in the community with respect. That was the hospital correcting itself.

That nurse's warning came just after I began to work at the hospital, which meant that the next five-year cycle would come toward the end of my time there. Although I didn't realize it then, I even recall the first hint that things were going wrong.

By that time, I was working with a third set of night nurses. The second changeover had gone much more smoothly than the first. As before, these new hires were just out of nursing school. But this time the nursing administration had learned a lesson. These new nurses were far more capable. Two had been honor students and one of those, I felt, could have breezed through medical school. Their orientation went better and, since not all the previous night nurses had moved to other shifts, the experience level remained high. For that I was grateful.

But something else was happening. About this time, the hospital's nurses were starting to claim that their work was getting harder because the children were sicker. Although coming up with a measure for patient difficulty isn't easy, there was truth to their claim. I know I was finding it harder to do the extras, including backing up nurses.

Looking back, though, I don't think that was because our kids were mysteriously getting sicker. There was no epidemic. Hem-Onc stayed full, but it was almost always full. Having more than one empty room was rare except around Christmas. Looking back, I suspect the reason lay with later arrivals and earlier discharges. The easiest Hem-Onc patients to care for were those who had yet to get treatment or those who about to go home. With those removed, the kids who remained would be sicker, bringing more work and greater stress.

Financial issues flowing from growing concern about rising medical costs may have been one reason, causing patients to be discharged earlier. But more important, at least for our Hem-Onc kids, was the opening of a Ronald MacDonald House a few blocks away. It was a great blessing. Our less sick kids could stay in a home-like setting and, if an emergency developed, be back in the hospital in minutes. They could stay in the House before treatment began and for a few days after their discharge. That partly explained the sicker kids on Hem-Onc. Ronald, bless his clownish heart, was taking care of those who were almost well.

That's the context for my first clue that something was amiss. One night, the nurse I was working with on Hem-Onc found herself with several exceptionally sick kids—more than she felt she could safely handle. Normally, the medical unit's three nurses each took one of our clusters of rooms, with the nurse on Hem-Onc having the fewest but sickest kids. But that night, to help the overburdened nurse, the other two nurses each took one or two of her more stable patients, allowing her to concentrate on the really sick. Having endured the disaster of the year before, I was delighted to see them handling this crisis so well. The better nurses did their job, the more manageable mine became.

Unfortunately, when the head nurse arrived at 6 a.m. she didn't see things that way. She didn't even consider the possibility they were right. When the nurses tried to explain that staff assignments made the day before were faulty, she attacked them for not doing their job properly. I was so ticked off by her attack that, while I didn't take on her directly—she and I were never on the best of terms—I did make a point of later telling the nurses that I felt they'd handled the crisis well.

At the time, I didn't attach much importance to the incident. I marked it down as the head nurse simply not liking the criticism implied by that night's too-heavy work load. She attacked those nurses to divert attention from herself. Besides, the clash itself was minor, and, even though I didn't care for that head nurse, I knew it wasn't easy to predict the next night's work load.

Slowly, however, other things happened that bothered me. Relations between the easy-going evening and the less experienced night nurses remained cordial. But relations between the younger night nurses and the decade-older day nurses became strained, particularly during change-of-shift reports. I wasn't involved in that clash myself. During morning report, I was busy making sure everything was well with the kids and their parents as they woke up. As few problems as possible had to be left for the next shift. But I heard enough to know what was happening wasn't fair.

During her eight-hour shift, a nurse has to make many decisions and some don't go well. Since most problems are minor and quickly corrected, that was rarely an issue. But some day nurses were making a big deal out of anything and linking minor mistakes or even the mere appearance of mistakes with gross incompetence. As a result, the night nurses I worked with were becoming touchy and irritable. They feared morning report, knowing that any little thing could trigger an attack. Since we were a team, when they got uptight, my job got harder.

Again I made excuses. At the time, I blamed the clashes on obvious differences between nurses on the two shifts. To myself, I described two of Hem-Onc's day nurses as "something that rhymes with witches." Rightly or wrongly, I suspected that only seniority had given them their positions. Not being talented, they hadn't moved into the specialty nursing slots that more capable nurses typically filled and loved. As a result, after about a decade at the hospital, they were doing the same work as recent nursing school graduates. That must have irked them, particularly since two new nurses were sharp and would obviously go far. I also suspected that only the lack of experience (and thus confidence) of these new nurses made them wither under attack. A year or two later, and those 'rhymes with witches' would not dare bully them.

Limited careers, I thought then, wasn't the only reason for these clashes. Another problem went beyond professional enmity and included woman-versus-woman envy. The two smart night nurses were also exceptionally pretty—I tend to notice such things. One was happily married. The other was single and had no trouble getting attention from the eligible bachelors among the residents. As Shakespeare put it, "Hell hath no fury like a woman spurned."

Competition like that was certainly real. I saw it at one of the evening nursing grand rounds. Arriving, I looked around at the 50 to 60 nurses there and was surprised at how well-dressed and properly made up they were. "That makes no sense," I thought to myself. "Why did they go to so much trouble to look good at a meeting when only other women would be attending?" I knew they hadn't dressed up to get my attention. They had no reason to even suspect I'd be there. This was clearly women intending to impress other women, perhaps suggesting that appearance plays a similar role among women that sports prowess and money does among men. "I look better than you," a woman is implicitly saying, "so if I'm interested in a guy, back off."

Looking back, I realize now that I was at least partially wrong about those 'rhymes with witches.' Yes, some had less than winsome personalities, and I remember being impressed that the plight of our sick and often dying children was sometimes able to wrench kindness even from their cold hearts. But that wasn't the whole story. The previous and far-less-capable wave of new nurses hadn't drawn this scorn, so why were they so critical of these talented new nurses? If I'd been thinking more clearly, I would have realized that something much more serious was happening. That dread five-year cycle had returned.

My Nights with Leukemia

36. Nurses Attacked

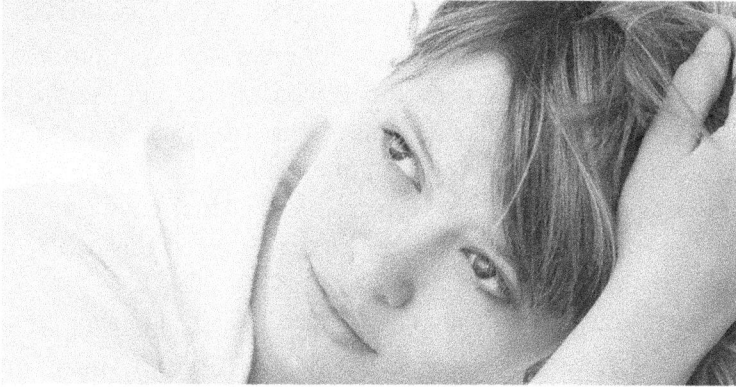

Normally, at the end of my shift, I walked the ten minutes back to my darkened basement apartment, fell into bed, and was sound asleep in a couple of minutes. With the exception of the staff crisis shortly after I started, no matter how bad the tensions were at the hospital, I no trouble sleeping. My body had learned to take sleep when it could. But this day was an exception because I taught a CPR class.

Just before going home, I dropped by the medical unit. As soon as the head nurse saw me, she pounced, fangs bare and claws drawn. She wanted to know why I'd left dirty sheets in a particular room. Since it wasn't my habit to do that, I couldn't answer. Like my earlier experience when that head nurse had attacked the night nurses for no good reason, I simply wrote it off as another illustration that she wasn't up to her job. Without any investigation, she'd attacked me.

That night I asked the nurse I'd been working with if she knew what had happened. She did. When I'd passed through at the end of shift, she'd been in the room with the boy, who had a tube running into his stomach to suction away gastric fluids. After I left, she moved him and a surge of stomach contents shot up the tube, with some spilling out a vent onto the sheets. If she'd told me, I'd have changed the sheets. But she hurried off to give report, fearing yet another encounter with those 'rhymes with witches.' One of the latter told the head nurse about the sheets without investigating. The head nurse then pounced on me.

At times, I get so ticked off about something that I don't want to talk about it. That's what happened with this incident. Without putting any pressure on my nurse, I suggested that she might want to tell the head nurse what'd happened. I didn't push, so I doubt she did. Otherwise, I let it pass. I felt that I had better things to do than get mixed up in hospital politics, particularly politics this stupid.

There's another revealing example. One day, the head nurse insisted that I stay over for a talk. She'd found what she thought was a fault in the care I'd been giving Jackie. You might remember that, to prevent problems during chemotherapy, we ran a sodium bicarbonate IV to keep our kids urine slightly alkaline, typically 6.5. Jackie's chemotherapy had began about midnight, she said, but I had not logged a urine PH for her until about 4 a.m.

I remembered the night well. Nothing about Jackie escaped my attention, so her chemotherapy was a momentous event. It meant my special little kid had recovered enough to finally start treatment. I also remembered why it took four hours to get that PH. I'd not been on duty for her previous diaper change. That about 2 a.m. had included a stool, which made the urine PH invalid. That 4 a.m. reading was the first I could take. I'd missed nothing.

Why didn't I raise an alarm about that lack of a reading? Because unlike that head nurse I knew my job. Much could go wrong when we gave chemotherapy. I've given some examples. But what did *not* go wrong was that alkaline PH. That we knew how to manage. The only exception came one evening when an evening nurse let a girl drink a glass of highly acidic cranberry juice. It took a couple of hours for her urine PH to recover. I know, because I was carefully watching it.

Besides, what could we have done to get an earlier reading? Remember, Jackie was a baby. We couldn't tell her to void like we might a child. True, we could have given her Lasix to force urination, but that would have interrupted her chemotherapy, a move so ridiculous, no one would have even considered it. No, I did all I could do—wait for that 4 a.m. diaper to get urine PH, well aware that it mattered. That PH, when it came, was fine. There was no problem.

Even worse was this head nurse's apparent ignorance about just how focused I was on Jackie's care. I never missed a urine PH for any child during my 16 months on Hem-Onc. I certainly wasn't going to slip up with the very patient I cared about the most. Every nurse on the medical unit knew how much Jackie meant to me, but our head nurse apparently didn't know that. That, I thought at the time, was odd.

Should I have handled both clashes differently? Even today, I'm not sure. That those attacks were malicious and unfair mattered. It showed that the bullying was expanding beyond day-nurse-on-night-nurse attacks into the administration. No one was safe, not even aides.

Her charges were so unfair, perhaps I should have met with the head of nursing and complained. When you take a clash with an immediate superior up the chain of command, it helps to have facts on your side, as I did here. Even those who have no intention of being fair can be intimidated into silence.

Others had similar experiences. Recently, I listened to an audio book on George Orwell as I showered. It was obvious that Orwell drew some of the horrors in his anti-utopian novel *1984* from his own terrible experiences in an English boarding school. Like the lead character in his famous novel, Orwell wasn't able to stop the abuse. The bad guys win in *1984*, in part, because Orwell didn't know how to stop bullying. But his biographer noted that another writer at his school at that time did find a solution. Bullied by one of the biggest guys at the school, he simply walked up to the guy and, without any warning, punched him in the face. Yes, today that's politically incorrect, but it's also true that neither that guy nor anyone else at the school ever bullied him again. Within every bully, beats the heart of a coward. Strike back, and he'll turn to softer targets.

Perhaps after discovering out how unfairly I'd been treated, I should have taken the matter directly to the head of nursing as a kind of verbal punch without warning. The best fight is one you can win, and those were clashes I could have won.

Such a move was also legitimate. For a clash with a head nurse, my only appeal was to the head of nursing. True, it wouldn't have stopped those dreadful day nurses from bullying the new night nurses, but it might have created a bubble of protection around me. "Mess with Mike, and you'll be sorry." Cue spooky music—I like that. If you ever have to live with unpleasant work or school politics, consider inflicting carefully thought out pain on the wrongdoers.

In a way, I would end up doing something like that as my parting gift to the nurses on the teen unit. I'll write more about that later. For now, we'll look at the what these growing clashes and the resulting tensions meant for those who should have mattered most, our sick children.

37. Aki's Overdose

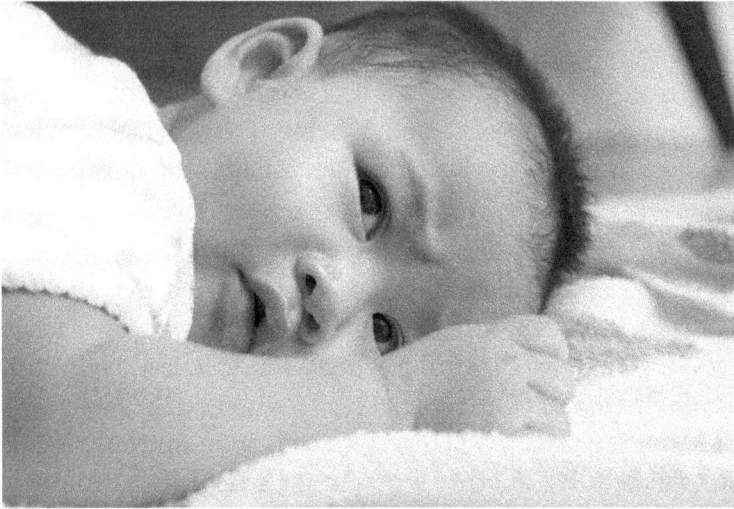

If I'd been smarter, I'd have know that a conflict this intense would not confine itself to a battle between shifts, with occasional ill-considered venom from the head nurse. The poison would eventually move inside shifts and even between the nurse and aide who normally worked amiably together as a team, sharing a common set of duties. That came for me one night when the nurse I was working with—the pretty, smart, single one—suddenly pounced on me.

Why had I wasted so much time, she demanded, staying with a boy whose temperature had to be taken rectally? I could have used the two-minute wait, she claimed, with some other patient. That was nonsense, I thought, but I got nowhere when I tried to explain that I never left a child with a rectal glass thermometer in his backside. The child might roll over and break it off, creating a horrible situation. I could have added that this kid, bless his bratty heart, might toss the thermometer on the floor, breaking it and scattering glass and mercury around the room. That meant a messy and time-consuming cleanup. Finally, I could have pointed out that boy was in isolation. Counting the time spent disrobing, leaving, re-robing and re-entering his room, I'd have saved mere seconds. Unfortunately, I was too angry to understand that it wasn't me that had her behaving so illogically. The two of us were getting sucked into that maelstrom of recrimination.

Another of her criticisms that night made even less sense. At the start of evening shift, she'd told me that she'd do the vital signs on an isolation patient. We normally got vital signs done by midnight, so at 12:30 a.m., when she still hadn't found time for the boy, I went in and did them for her. That was of little importance. The boy wasn't so sick that he needed nurse-only attention, and that night I had time to spare. I even thought I was doing her a favor. Unfortunately, she didn't react that way. More trouble and yet another attack. Sigh, and we normally got along so well. Teamwork was collapsing.

Worst of all was her third attack. That mattered most because she was right. Our younger kids slept in high-sided cribs so they would not climb out and fall. To do anything, you had to lower one side and remember to raise it back up before you left. Doing otherwise was a big no-no. Distracted by my clashes with her, for one child I forgot to raise the crib side back up. Nothing happened, but she saw it open and pounced on me for a third time. That was the only time in over two years I made that mistake, so it was easy to see what was happening. The growing unpleasantness was affecting how well I did my job and putting our kids at risk.

In that nurse's favor, near the end of the shift she told me that morning she was facing her first three-month review as a nurse. Hearing that, I understood why she'd been so tense and ill-tempered. Her anger at me was an extension of her fears about that review. That was also why my well-meant effort to pick up work she was slow to do only made matters worse. It made her look bad and, feeling insecure, she struck out. Unfortunately, clashes like that were now common. She and I were in the middle of a civil war.

By this point, the unit's morale was terrible. The default mode was to criticize to protect yourself. Risking another "Not Done" lecture, I made a bold attempt steer everyone's thoughts back to what mattered. I took pictures of many of our kids, and, in the wee hours of the night with no head nurse around, I posted them near the entrance, offering copies, at cost, to parents and staff. And no, I didn't ask for permission. After all, I told myself, it was a blank wall, why not use it? In the end, I was protected by the popularity of the pictures.

Unfortunately, those photos weren't enough to reverse our troubles. Our troubles were far beyond where anything I did mattered. Something far worse than clashes between staff was about to happen.

The patient was Aki, a two-year-old boy with a lung tumor. I'd taken care of him on a previous visit and had gotten to know his parents, who were from Japan but living in Anchorage, Alaska. His symptoms had grown worse, so just after admission, a resident had written up an order for IV morphine to control his pain. And no, I never saw the order. But I know it must have been a resident because no regular physician would have been that stupid. The dose for that little boy—who've never received morphine before—was far too large. Later we discovered there'd been a power-of-ten mistake. This small boy got a hefty adult dose. An experienced physician would have known at a glance that was wrong. Even more chilling, so would a nurse who wasn't under unusual stress.

That night we would have almost certainly killed that little boy but for a most fortunate happenstance. His IV morphine began about 1 a.m., when most parents would have been asleep in a darkened room. But his parents had just flown in from Alaska and were still on Anchorage time, two hours earlier than our own. They were up and the lights were on in their room when their son suddenly stopped breathing and turned blue—classic signs of a morphine overdose.

Matters quickly got worse. The narcotics cabinet was supposed to have Narcan, which counters a narcotic overdose in seconds. It wasn't there, having been removed a couple years earlier due to thefts. Fortunately, we were only a few hundred feet away from the pharmacy, so someone ran for Narcan. Little Aki was saved, but just barely.

As nursing staff, we knew this should never have happened and that we were partly to blame. I overheard the shift supervisor telling the boy's nurse something she should have known. "You need to memorize the usual doses for the common medications for the ages of children you care for," the supervisor said. "And when you see a medical order that's outside that range, question it."

That's what usually happened. One example was a similar mistake months earlier. Around 2 a.m., the pharmacist on duty called, wanting me to check a medication order. We had the original, while what he had was a sometimes hard-to-read carbon copy. After I confirmed the dose, he said, "Well this drug isn't very toxic, so it must be OK."

When the drug, an antibiotic, arrived, the nurse and I knew something was wrong. Antibiotics typically came in one or two small glass bottles. This dose was ten bottles in a large plastic bag. Given at 4 a.m., it'd take until almost 8 a.m., when the next dose was due, to run it in.

That made no sense. The doctor who'd written the order was awakened and his mistake discovered. He taken the amount to be given over 24 hours and applied it to one four-hour dose.

Why did a nurse catch the antibiotic overdose but not that for morphine? Yes, in part, that was due to the ridiculous look of all those bottles. Even a large dose of morphine came from a single bottle, so an overdose wasn't as obvious. But it's also true that a nurse who wasn't under extreme pressure would look at any morphine order carefully. Morphine can kill.

But the ultimate cause of this almost-lethal mistake was the unhealthy pressure on our nurses. That mistake was like my failing to raise that crib railing. Someone who's anxious and fearful, particularly of unfair attacks, doesn't think as well as someone whose is confident of support and trust. Fear addles your brain and anxiety makes you stupid.

That overdose was the final straw. Something destructive was going on. Personal attacks were common, tensions were high, and morale was plummeting. Even worse, mistakes were being made that could kill. Not knowing what I could do and having failed with the one attempt I'd made, I felt I had to get away.

I was also worn out after sixteen months on night shift. I'd worked nights, mostly on Hem-Onc, with three sets of nurses, and even those in the third set were now moving to other shifts. The nursing student I'd worked with had graduated and was gone. Almost all the 30-some aides I'd started with had left. I'd endured much and needed a change.

When a day position opened up on the teen unit, I took it. The good part was that I wouldn't be leaving cancer patients behind. On Hem-Onc we'd cared for children with cancer up their tenth birthday. After that, the teen unit handled every kind of teen problem, including cancers. I'd see fewer leukemia patients, but more with bone cancers along with major orthopedic surgeries.

Perhaps most important of all, from floating to the teen unit, I had friends among the nurses there. Nothing they said suggested that these dangerous clashes had spread there. At the time, they seemed confined to our unit, perhaps being driven by our ill-tempered head nurse and those 'rhymes with witches' nurses. For a time, that would seem to be true.

And as you will see, on the teen unit I would discover a new sort of patient and new challenges.

38. Adapting to Teens

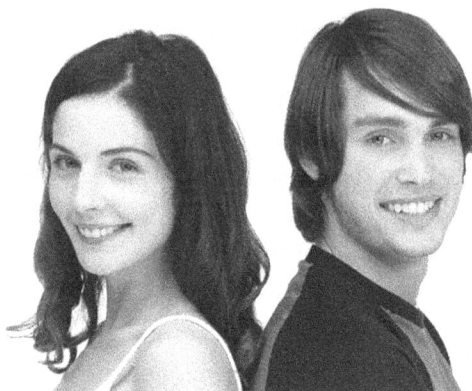

On night shift, I'd occasionally floated to the teen unit on the second floor, so I knew what it meant when I transferred there—a seeming overabundance of patients. During days and evenings, the teen unit had a patient-to-nurse ratio of about twelve to one, already greater than the ten to one I'd experienced with the younger kids on the medical unit, and almost twice the seven to one ratio on Hem-Onc.

At night there were only two nurses for teens, so when I floated there the nurse/patient ratio was about seventeen-to-one, something I found overwhelming. I had to constantly consult my patient card to remember which teen had what illness. Even worse, if an emergency required all the attention of the other nurse and aide, my nurse and I would suddenly find ourselves responsible for almost three dozen teens. Of course, some of that fretting was psychological. I wasn't used to juggling so many patients, but that didn't mean it wasn't possible.

There was also the familiarity factor. On Hem-Onc, I could get to know my patients well, sometimes caring for them for months at a time. We typically had no more than one or two new kids admitted over the space of a week. But when I floated to the teen unit for a night, all seventeen kids were new. As a result, I did not know who needed extra attention and who didn't. I muddled through by depending on my nurse. My float complete, I was glad to return to the more familiar Hem-Onc—that is until I made the move to teens permanent.

What struck me most about my new assignment was the wide variety of illnesses that I must now handle. The teen unit dealt with what in younger children was taken care of by three units: medical, surgical, and psychiatric. It handled almost every sort of illness for those ten and over. The only exceptions were the ICU, for those in fragile condition, and Rehab, for those with major disabilities such as quadriplegia. Both needed nurse-to-patient ratios of two- or four-to-one.

The mix of illnesses also changed. Small kids have numerous infections, hence those 'poopers and croupers' isolation rooms. With teens, trauma was more common. For kids, life-threatening illnesses involved the blood—leukemia and aplastic anemia. With teens, I saw bone cancer for the first time. I still remember caring for a sixteen-year-old girl whose left arm had been amputated at the elbow. That shocked me, because I'd always associated missing arms or legs with men who'd gone to war.

My greatest frustration, however, came from moving from Hem-Onc, a specialized care unit, to a part of the hospital where, quite frankly, the nurses saw so many different kinds of illnesses, they didn't get a chance to become good at caring for some of them.

Psychiatric problems were common, as were orthopedic surgeries. For psychiatric problems, we were baby sitters, sending them off for their appointments, so our lack of expertise mattered little. On the other hand, back surgeries were so common, we knew how to handle them well. At that time, orthopedic surgeries were so much a part of what the hospital did, that Orthopedic was part of its name. You can read more about them and the issues they created in *Hospital Gowns*.

Unfortunately—and despite its life-threatening seriousness—leukemia was woefully neglected on the teen unit. On the medical unit, we'd typically have at least five or six kids with leukemia any one time. All the night nurses worked on Hem-Onc and all learned how to handle their care. With teens, the opposite was true. Patients with leukemia were less common, we rarely had more than one at a time, and many nurses had little experience caring for them.

As a result, the nurses often did what I do when faced with something I don't understand, they faked it based on what they did know. In one situation, a boy with leukemia was to get radiation for a bone marrow transplant. Every nurse on the medical unit would have known that meant transport to the large cancer center for whole body radiation. Even more important, every nurse would know that was an extraordinary step. The dose was lethal and, if the transplant didn't take, the child would die in a few weeks. When you're doing something that serious, you want to be competent and professional. You don't want to look like an idiot.

But when this boy's nurse heard he was to get radiation that morning, she assumed that meant a nearby university hospital, where almost all our other radiation treatments were given, and she tried to arrange transportation there. The boy's parents had to argue with her to get the situation corrected. When I heard that, I gritted my teeth. Not good.

Even more telling, it wasn't that nurse's fault. Fewer leukemia patients meant much less of what we had in abundance on Hem-Onc—expertise built on experience. That could have been corrected by regular, systematic training, but frighteningly little about leukemia was being taught to these nurses, must less the brave new world of bone marrow transplants. A few sessions required of all teen nurses would have helped. Formal training was lagging. I'll say more about that later.

Even more disturbing was a situation that arose toward the end of my time at the hospital when the teen unit's head nurse returned after a leave of absence. The feeling that leukemia patents weren't receiving enough specialized attention had been growing, which was good. But when she brought up her solution, I felt like screaming "No!"

At that time, for kids ten and under the hospital had Hem-Onc, a specialized set of rooms just for them. In a clumsy sort of way, the head nurse seemed to be thinking that our teen unit also needed rooms set aside just for them, as if separate rooms were all that mattered. But what made me angry was that she wanted kids with leukemia to be mixed with those with cystic fibrosis. "You idiot!" I felt like yelling. "Don't your realize, that this would place teens with almost no immune system (leukemia) close to teens whose many lung infections mean they're often carrying bacteria that's resistant to most antibiotics (cystic fibrosis)?" Often, only an effective antibiotic stood between a child with leukemia and death. Fortunately, I knew enough to not worry. Our Hem-Onc doctors would squelch that idea in an instant. Still, it was disturbing to be working under a head nurse whose judgment was so poor.

There is good news. Since I worked there, cancer treatment has been reorganized. Leukemia patients, whatever their age, are now treated by a specialized Hem-Onc team. Care that critical needs specialized nursing care. It shouldn't be a side show. It should never get lost in the confusion of caring for all sorts of illnesses.

My Nights with Leukemia

39. Dreaded Politics

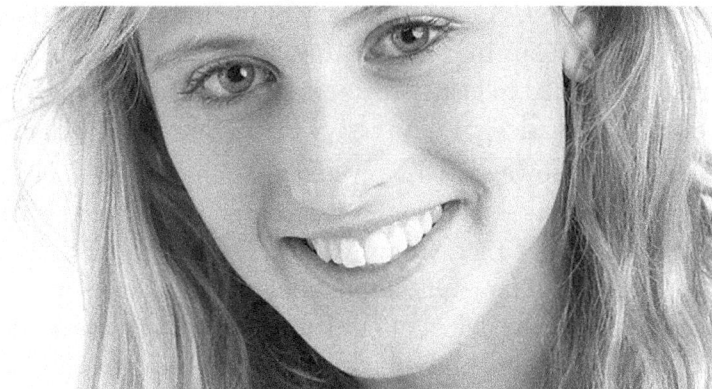

One change with my move to days with teens struck me more forc-
ibly than any other. That was hospital politics. At night there was
almost no politics. A nurse and I could live under the happy illusion that
we were running this state-of-the-art hospital. After all, no one came
around to challenge what we were doing. The hundreds of physicians,
administrators, and other staff who flooded into the building during the
day were for us little more than ghosts. During the day, those shadowy
figures busied themselves with creating little scraps of paper to keep us
occupied during the long nights when we ran the show.

Of course, that also meant that what we were to do was fixed from
the start of a shift. Only when a crisis arose did the situation at the end
of a shift differ from that at the start. The chief reason was the absence
of 'real' doctors. During my sixteen-months working nights, I never
saw the hospital's senior physicians. As a teaching hospital, at nights
the medical profession was represented by residents. They did deal with
emergencies and wrote up orders that we followed. But even the most
capable of them knew they were in training, so they rarely surprised
us. After a few months, I knew the routine, including any orders they
might write. I also knew that, for anything out of the ordinary, they'd
call their superiors.

In fact, it was easy to feel sorry for residents. These unfortunates, enduring their 32-hours shifts, could not even control their sleep. Through
the hospital's telephone operator, a nurse or I could hunt them down,
wake them up, and make them come to us. Even their ability to dis-

rupt what we did was minor. I worried constantly that some sleepy, bone-headed resident would issue a foolish or dangerous order when I was present, but I never saw that happen and, if one had, the nurse or I would have protested. Also, in the back of my mind lay the picture of a time each day, perhaps in mid-morning, when the residents, trembling from head to toe, had to justify their decisions during the night. By then I'd be home sound asleep. I didn't envy them. Better them than me.

On day shift, however, I discovered that change was constant and unrelenting. Doctors—real ones—darted in, issued new orders, and darted out. On top of that, we were always admitting and discharging patients. On nights, Hem-Onc admissions and discharges were so rare I don't recall a single one. Most of our late-night admissions on the medical unit as a whole were children who developed croup at bedtime.

On days, among my dozen teens there might be two discharges and as many admissions in eight hours. With teens, the hospital had good reason to discharge early. We were stuffed. During the ten months I worked there, we ran a near-constant 104% of capacity. One multi-bed room had enough extra space for an teen boy who was unlikely to need oxygen or suction.

That meant we were very busy and that sometimes led to amusing situations. One day we had a nursing student preparing for the following day when she would have one patient to care for. Yes, one. To me that seemed like a joke. Since the nurse and I were splitting a dozen kids between us, I had to force myself not to laugh at how seriously she was about deciding who that one would be.

Of course, I wanted her to take one my busier patients. The teenaged boy who'd accidentally shot himself with a shotgun, leaving a fist-sized exit wound, would have made a good choice. He was partially paralyzed, his wound required watching, and his dressings needed changing daily. But I also knew that this twenty-year-old girl might feel a little squeamish about caring for a boy only a few years younger than she, so I wasn't surprised that all the charts spread out in front of her were for girls. In *Hospital Gowns*, I write in great detail about the hidden role that embarrassment plays in medical care. This was an example.

The main problem lay with her choice of a girl. I suggested she pick one with serious problems, warning that otherwise she might find her patient discharged. She wouldn't listen. Instead, she picked an easy patient and began to study her chart. An order came for that girl to be discharged. Again, I suggested someone serious. Again she picked someone safe. Another order came, and that girl was also leaving. Necessity finally forced her to take someone who was actually sick, to my great relief. But she'd wasted time that, as a student, she could ill afford.

That said, I do understand what was going on. At first, working with hospitalized patients can be terrifying. "What if I do something stupid and someone dies?" But in a hospital, you can't play it safe. Circumstances will arise when someone's life may hinge on your good judgment. That comes with the job. You do your best and hope.

Day shift did have an advantage. With orders being issued by more experienced doctors, there was less reason to regard them with skepticism. That said, it was also harder to evade dubious orders. Two cases illustrate that.

On morning, an order came for Kay, a teen girl with cystic fibrous, to be given her vitamin K via IV rather than her usual pill. Her nurse fretted about that, recalling something about a potential for an adverse reaction. She was right. Drugs.com warns that IV-given vitamin K can cause "severe reactions, including fatalities." I'm afraid I wasn't helpful, merely observing that it seemed odd that an IV vitamin would be dangerous when a pill wasn't. (That's why I left medications to nurses.) Then I left for lunch. When I returned half-an-hour later, the unit was still recovering from the girl's severe reaction. Fortunately, the nurse had been prepared for that ill-advised order.

I faced a similar situation when two doctors examined a new admission with a skin infection and ordered Respiratory Isolation (mask and gown). That made no sense, and I was concerned about a nearby patient who was immunocompromised. I decided to meddle as quietly as possible. I called the hospital's infection control nurse, who agreed that the isolation should be Skin and Wound (mask, gown and gloves). Fortunately, the hospital's rules allowed her issue an order that superseded that of the now-departed doctors. I told the nurse the new order as casually as I could, so she could write it up. Then I changed the sign and put a box of gloves at the entrance. The teen with a weak immune system was now safe.

Yes, you've heard right. Despite my complaints about day politics, I was playing games myself, getting an order I liked to override one I didn't. Those doctors looked so harried, I told myself, they'll probably never notice. But if they had noticed and raised a fuss, some unpleasantness might have followed. Feathers would have flown, most of them mine, and the infectious control nurse and my nurse would have been drawn into the dispute. Hospital politics can be nasty.

Sadly, there are people on day shift who live for such squabbles. Trouble makes them feel more important. That's why I liked nights. It was easier to shape events without a fuss. The rules were relaxed and rebellion less unlikely to be noticed. Even if we were spotted, bureaucratic action was hobbled. What were these administrators going to do—ask us to stay over *with pay* to meet with them? Hardly punishment.

Here's a tip you might find handy if you find yourself working in a hospital. I made a point of being so good at what I was doing that I could, at times, evade stupid rules in the interests of my patients. If caught, it was easier to feign ignorance rather than admit willfulness. Something might be written up in my file, but there'd be more than enough good reviews to counter that. I'd learned that in college ROTC, where it was easier to earn a few extra merits sorting uniforms, than to fret over demerits from poorly polished shoes. I never learned to give my shoes the sort of shine that was expected.

One incident illustrates my working around a sometimes broken system. One day, a teen boy desperately needed an item from the laundry that we didn't have. I checked in Central Supply, and they were out, so I headed for my old unit where, just as I'd hoped, they had it in stock. As I departed with my loot, one of the 'rhymes with witches' nurses screamed at me that I shouldn't be doing that. Each department, she shouted, was billed for its laundry. I could care less. I had a patient in need, and that's what mattered. I'd stolen from the teen unit on more than a few nights when necessity demanded. This merely balanced the books. If the hospital wanted more precision in its accounting, it needed a procedure for borrowing.

Yes, nights were much better. Then, hospital politics meant little more than an occasional ill-tempered remark from a head nurse grumpy at the start of her day. Anything more, such as investigations and formal meetings, were simply too much trouble when the offenders worked nights—that is on the rare occasions when what happened at night even reached the ears of administrators. Like the old saying, "What happens in Vegas stays in Vegas," what happened on nights tended to stay on nights. Only problems really needing attention were passed on to days during the nurse's reports or as incident reports. That I liked.

Here's an illustration of just how different nights were. Among the first set of nurses I worked with was one whose husband was an officer on a Coast Guard cutter. He'd just returned from a long cruise, so she was spending her days with him rather than sleeping. One night she was particularly tired, so just after the 4 a.m. meds, she told me she'd be napping during her break. I thought no more about that. The kids were stable, and I had enough to keep me busy. But when the head nurse arrived at 6 a.m. I thought, "Oh no, she's not back yet!" Thinking quickly, I quietly slipped over to the cluster next to Hem-Onc and asked its nurse to listen out for anything. Then I began hunting for my nurse.

Fortunately, Sleeping Beauty was in the first place I looked, the nursing locker room. I woke her and hurried back. She followed a couple of minutes later, and it was all I could do to avoid bursting out laughing. It's hard to awake from two hours of sound sleep without showing it. Fortunately, the head nurse didn't realize what'd happened. Sometimes her cluelessness was a benefit.

In short, working with those teens, I soon learned that night shift and day shift were as different as night and day, and that, all things considered, I preferred the former. My body didn't like working nights, but my mind and personality clearly prefer the greater freedom and wider responsibilities of a hospital at night.

40. Still More Issues

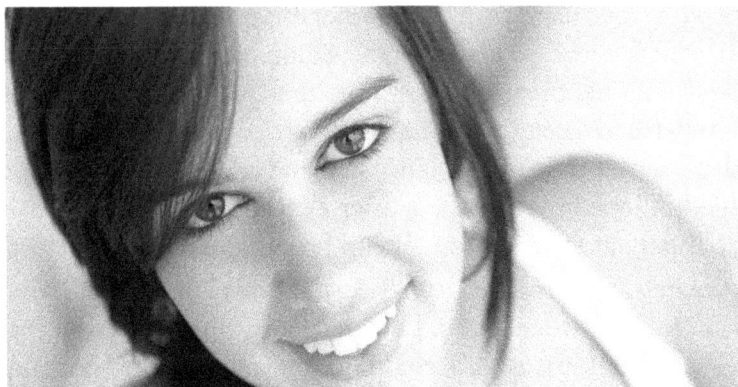

Further complicating my move to days with teens was a dramatic shift in how I related to these older patients. Win a small child's trust by being kind and gentle, and your difficulties were over. They trust you and with them trust is crucial. Having earned their friendship, I could focus on medical care rather than child psychiatry.

As any parent of a teen knows, the same isn't true of adolescents. They have issues piled on top of issues weighed down by still more issues. One room had so many problems, the nurse I worked with referred to it as a "psych ward." One of the four girls saw things that weren't there. Another ate so little, she was mere skin and bones. The third had troubles I've since forgotten.

Surprisingly, the one girl in the room who was emotionally together was the one with the most reasons to be a basket case. Cindy been so badly abused as a child that even at fifteen she was still undergoing corrective surgery. Fortunately, as a baby she'd been adopted by a kind and loving family. She was an absolute delight, and on her own initiative, she worked wonders with the other three. I still have a photo taken when I took her and her mother down to their car to go home.

The teens I had the most difficulty understanding were three girls being treated at various times for anorexia. All were exceptionally pretty and yet so troubled by fears of becoming fat that they ate almost nothing. Typically, for lunch they'd order skim milk and a green salad without dressing. We were under strict orders to never talk with them about food, which was good. Looking from their emaciated bodies to a tray almost devoid of calories, I felt like screaming, "Don't be crazy! Eat! You need more than this!" Sigh! I don't think I'd make a good psychiatrist. Too blunt and direct.

Anorexia was frustrating because there was no magic pill. At times it seemed that we were merely a pricey hotel to make their appointments with a psychiatrist more convenient—as well as to deal with that terrible time when their mental problem might become a life-threatening medical emergency. Reading about the treatment for anorexia today, little seems to have changed. What's wrong lies in how they view their bodies. It's a long struggle to get them to see themselves differently.

Other teens could be stubborn, particularly the boys. Part of post-op care for surgical patients was getting them to cough and deep breathe to reduce their chance of catching pneumonia. For that, I could show them the trick of holding a pillow to their chest to make coughing less painful, but since the boys were often as big as I am or bigger, my only real motivational tool was to be stubborner than they were, making it clear that I'd nag them until they complied with the surgeon's orders.

In every case but one that worked. The exception was a fool. As a boy of about six, he had drank Drano, doing enormous damage to his mouth and upper throat. Fifteen years later, he was still undergoing corrective surgeries. You'd think he'd have learned from all that, but he hadn't. Nothing I did could get him to cough and deep breathe. Not surprisingly, he developed pneumonia, lengthening his stay.

Working with teens also had benefits. There was no need to talk down to them. I could treat these almost-adults as if they were almost adults. When one boy was watching *The Wizard of Oz* where the munchkins celebrate the death of the wicked witch, I hinted to him that there were people at the hospital who made me want to sing: "Ding Dong! The Witch is dead. Which old Witch? The Wicked Witch! Ding Dong! The Wicked Witch is dead." No four-year-old would have understood what I meant.

My humor can be weird. When girls were reading *Seventeen* magazine, I would sometimes put on a frown and try to convince them that the magazine's name must be taken seriously. As mere fifteen- or sixteen-year-olds, I would say with mock seriousness, they had no right to read *Seventeen*, in fact the hospital banned such reading.

Alas, they didn't understand, and years later I think I understand why. As a member of the hospital staff, they expected what I said to be literal and factual—"drink this and do that" orders. My not-to-be-taken-seriously humor floated over their heads. A nurse I once dated understood that. She told me I was "facetious," meaning that I find humor in making remarks that aren't meant to be taken seriously but often are. Alas, those teen girls, otherwise so adorable, did take me seriously and drew a blank. They'd stare at me when they should have laughed.

Teens were also different in ways that were important legally as well as medically. They were at or were approaching the age when they could make their own treatment decisions. That could be good or bad.

In one case, a seventeen-and-a-half year old girl was admitted with leukemia. Her exact age mattered both medically and legally. Medically, at that age her chance of being cured was much less than that for a small child. Legally, her treatment was complicated by the fact that her family belonged to a religion that opposes blood transfusions. Not being able to give blood products meant that her chemotherapy would have to be far less aggressive and more likely to fail.

At this point, keep in mind that people in that particular religion have done us a great service. Many court decisions about the right to refuse care involve them. In general, unattached adults can refuse even basic, life-saving care such as a transfusion, but parents of small children can't refuse for either themselves or their children. In both cases, a minor will suffer, so that child's welfare trumps religious objections.

This girl's situation was complicated by the fact that she was just six months shy of eighteen, when she would be able to decide for herself. As I heard the story, the doctors involved decided not to contest the girl's decision not to receive transfusions. There was no time for delay. Her treatment must start quickly and, if successful, it wouldn't be completed until she was eighteen. Going to court would have delayed treatment and created a painful mess.

The result was a muddle. I recall going into her room, where she was invariably surrounded by her family. "Where do you draw the line," I thought to myself, "between her family supporting her decision to refuse blood and their applying so much pressure that she can make no choice of her own." I never found an answer. Rightly or wrongly, the weakened chemotherapy wasn't enough. Her diagnosis, treatment, and death all came during my ten months on the teen unit. The only saving grace was that at least the treatment she did receive was less harsh and in the end the outcome might have been the same.

41. UNEXPECTED TRAGEDIES

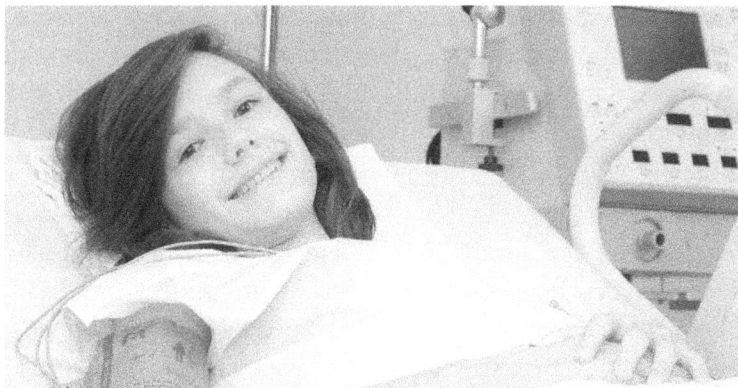

When you're handling patients, there's a big difference between carrying for someone who dies after a long and well-understood illness and someone who arrives suddenly and under a cloud of mystery, dying within hours. The first fits the medical model well. Sickness is followed by diagnosis and treatment, while death comes after the treatment fails. All that is as it should be, orderly and predictable. The scientific passion for cause and effect is satisfied.

In the second situation, however, the time line of events gets crushed almost beyond recognition. Diagnosis hasn't been completed or treatment even begun before death intervenes, putting an end to all human action. With an auto accident, that's easy to accept. A powerful external force has intervened and taken someone's life. What's harder to accept is a situation where someone arrives at the hospital well enough to walk to their bed and talk with staff and yet dies suddenly, often without a diagnosis beyond that which led to their initial admission and with no treatment worthy of the name.

I've already described Ralph, who arrived with an extremely low platelet count and in an advanced stage of leukemia (as I remember it). There the mystery lay only in my perception. I hadn't taken care of him before and neither had anyone else on our unit. He was new to us, but not to medical care. His diagnosis and extensive treatment had taken place elsewhere. Our confusion came because our perception of his death didn't fit our expectation that children admitted for the first time should live at least a few months rather than die within hours.

Working with teens, on one occasion I experienced that same crushed time line in a way that, to this day, leaves me mystified, with more questions than answers. The patient was Tammy, a girl of about fourteen with the usual chatty, outgoing, people-centered personality of someone with Down syndrome. I took care of her admission, and she certainly livened up the room she shared with three other teen girls. She had a captive audience and loved it.

Like Ralph, Tammy had been admitted with a low platelet count. That in itself wasn't unusual. They'd been common on Hem-Onc. What was unusual was the admonition that came with her admission. We were to do everything we could to assist the family's physician, who would be playing a major role in her treatment. No other patient I cared for ever came with that stipulation. Patients came to us because their treatment was beyond the resources of family physicians. Those doctors needed to be kept informed, but they rarely played a role.

The next day, for reasons I've since forgotten, the cluster of rooms that included Tammy's was split between two aides. I was assigned the multi-bed boys' room next to hers, along with several private rooms, but not her multi-bed room. At report, we were told she'd been given a sedative to keep her calm. Excitement isn't good in someone with a platelet count as low as hers. Unfortunately, the pill hadn't calmed her. She was so delighted by her roommates, I could hear her chatting away from the hall. At the time I smiled. At least she's enjoying being here.

About 8:30 that morning, the other girls in her room called out. Tammy had quit talking and was sitting up in bed, staring blankly ahead. A code was called, and she was transported to the ICU, but it was too late. She was dead, I assume of a stroke, less than a day after being admitted and before any formal diagnosis.

I was left confused. Keep in mind that a low platelet count is a medical 'sign' rather than a diagnosis. It has many causes. At the time I wondered if she had leukemia. Children with Down syndrome, I knew, are more likely to get leukemia. Today, we also know that children with Down actually respond better to treatment than other children, but I'm not sure that was known then. Could that be the mystery? Did Tammy have leukemia? We were told that the mother was very attached to the daughter. Could breaking the bad news slowly be why the family doctor was involved?

Maybe and yet that makes little sense. Almost all the children we cared for had parents who loved them deeply. Family doctors showed no hesitation in telling those parents that their child had leukemia before sending the child to us. Nor did our specialists delay that awful news. The sooner a diagnosis was explained, the sooner treatment could begin.

That's why for me the woefully incomplete tale of chatty young Tammy will forever remain a mystery. In life, some stories have no clear plot and no happy ending.

Finally, although it doesn't involve a death, there's one more mysterious tragedy that I should mention because, as terrible as it was, it provided the answer to a question that had long troubled me.

In *Hospital Gowns*, I mention Kate, a slender girl in her early twenties, to illustrate how difficult it was for staff to know what to say when the hospital itself blunders badly. She came to us for heart surgery, one in a series she'd been having since she was a child. I did the admission workup for her one afternoon. The next morning she went for her operation, transferring to the ICU afterward.

About a week later, Kate returned to us, with much of what had happened to her shrouded in guilt and mystery. We were told little more than that the sodium bicarbonate she was being given through her IV had leaked into her lower arm, causing serious tissue damage. Imagine someone with a lower arm as grey as slate. That's how terrible it looked. It was most sickening.

Since Kate was again my patient, I wasn't satisfied with the little I'd been told at report and turned to her medical chart, which should have told all. If something like that happened again, I wanted to be ready. Alas, I found absolutely nothing in her chart. On one page, all was going well post-op. On the next, it was clear that something had gone terribly wrong, but no details were given.

Why the silence? Because everything in that chart was evidence that could be used in court. Given the serious harm done to the girl and the fact that her father was an attorney, there would almost certainly be a lawsuit. Given how chatty doctors usually are in those charts, behind that silence I sensed the baneful influence of the hospital's lawyer.

That experience, grim as it was, led to a startling revelation. You might recall that, from my early months at the hospital, I'd been asking myself how I could change a medical situation that I felt was putting a patient in danger. Recall that by that I meant real power not just the ability to persuade others. I wanted to be able to say, "This is wrong and must change," and have the phones of some very important people begin to ring whatever the time, day or night.

Kate's charts, incomplete as they were, gave me the answer I'd been seeking for so long. While it was true that those charts were typically used by doctors to communicate among themselves, they were open to all staff. I had used them to describe events only I had seen—such as a seizure.

I now had my answer. In a crisis, I would tell those around me that, if my concerns weren't taken seriously, I would place them in the patient's medical chart. There they'd become legal evidence that could not be concealed. With that warning, the hospital would become legally culpable for what followed. As a legal dictionary notes, *culpable* means "sufficiently responsible for criminal acts or negligence to be at fault and liable for the conduct. Sometimes culpability rests on whether the person realized the wrongful nature of his/her actions and thus should take the blame."

Creating culpability by charting my concerns meant the hospital could no longer tell the news media or a courtroom, "But we didn't realize this might happen." They had been warned, so they knew. Using hospital security to keep me from that chart would make no difference. I could always find a lawyer and draw up a sworn and dated statement.

Even more surprisingly, as odd as it sounds, what I was doing would transform my greatest weakness—my lowly place in the hospital hierarchy—into my greatest asset. "An aide was able to spot this problem," a courtroom lawyer could say, "so why were the hospital's physicians so blind?" In general, I dislike lawyers. But in some situations they can be invaluable.

Yes, what I was contemplating was extremely high risk. If later events proved me wrong, it might cost my job. But, as I often reminded myself, I could always get another job. I couldn't give a child back her life.

Finally, keep in mind that I'd only take that step in exceptional circumstances. During the 26 months I worked at the hospital, I never faced a problem I couldn't get changed by lesser means. Persuasion is almost always better than threats.

Next, we look at patients who were in comas and how that crude diagnosis often masks very different situations.

My Nights with Leukemia

42. Differing Comas

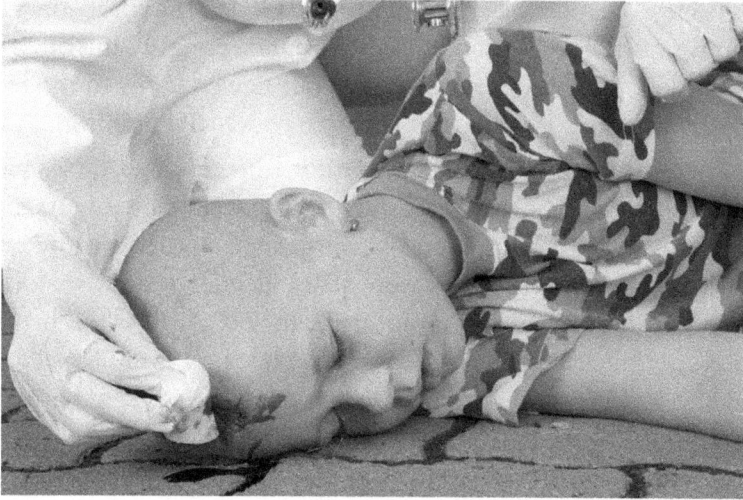

Iknew about comas even before I transferred to work with teens. I'd taken care of a boy named Sam who was in a deep coma. I once had a picture of him being held by a nurse, one in which he seems to be looking at the camera. He isn't. His eyes were open and looking out, but they weren't looking at anything, and they didn't focus or follow movement. They simply looked in one direction. In kindness, the nurse who was holding him had oriented his eyes toward the camera.

Sam was about two-years old, a handsome little black boy who must have had an adventurous spirit. His coma came from a terrible accident. At his mother's apartment building, he'd wandered off and fallen face down into a shallow wading pool. Perhaps knocked out by the fall, he'd lain face down in the water for some fifteen minutes.

The critical factor wasn't his time in the water. I also took care of Harold, a boy of about six, who'd been drown for some 45 minutes before being found. Sam had been left severely brain-damaged and was with us for at least two months. Harold stayed overnight night for observation and recovered with nothing more that serious than an odd twitch. The critical factor was water temperature. Sam had drown in the warm water of a wading pool. Harold had drown in the cold water of a lake and was protected by a reflex that's particularly strong in children and that reduces the brain's oxygen consumption when the face is immersed in cold water.

In the end, Sam died from a tragic miscalculation. He'd grown stable enough—if anyone in a coma that deep can be called stable—that he was to go home in a few days. Without thinking through the implications, his classification was changed to No Code. That probably made it easier to sign off on the discharge his parents were insisting on. The No Code then led, by a train of impeccable but flawed logic, to the removal of his heart monitor. If you're not going to code, why monitor?

But there was still a reason to monitor him. He had a tracheotomy that required cleaning every few hours. In the wee hours of one night, it became clogged with mucus, and he suffocated. When I came on duty the following night, the nurses were still talking about how shaken up his nurse that night was. No monitor meant no alarm when he choked and could not breathe. When she went to check on him, it was too late. All the implications of that No Code had not been thought through.

Later, when I was working with teens, traumas seemed a more common cause of comas. One day I received a call to go to Admissions and transport a 14-year-old comatose boy to our floor. As I went to pick him up, I thought, "This makes no sense. Comatose people come in through the ER with a lot of fuss and bother."

Actually, it made perfect sense. Jeff was from our area but had been with his family on vacation on the Oregon coast. He'd been riding a dirt bike over sand dunes when one jump had gone awry, leaving him in a coma with several broken bones. Two months at a hospital in Oregon had healed his broken bones, but he was still in a coma. So he could come home, someone at his family's church had loaned a recreational vehicle as a quasi-ambulance. A nurse volunteered to manage his IV during the long drive north.

Jeff's coma was nothing like Sam's. Often, he would turn his eyes toward me and focus, giving the impression that he could see me. I was even told that there had been a few times when he had spoken. At least some of the time he may have been in a 'locked in' state, aware of his surroundings but unable to communicate.

Sam had gone through sleep and wake cycles but little else. Jeff behaved in ways that went well beyond waking and sleeping. Once every few days, he would become upset, tensing his muscles, breathing fast, and having an extremely rapid heart rate. He wasn't on a heart monitor, so I couldn't count his heart beats until a nurse showed me a trick. Count very fast in your head, she said, and then mesh that rate with the beating of his heart. Count for five seconds and multiply by twelve. That worked. His heart was pounding 180 times a minute or three times a second. Those upsets added to my suspicion that he knew what was happening around him. When his mother was there, she was much more successful at calming him than I was.

Jeff's story ends tragically. We could do little for him, so his family established a network of friends to care for him at home. A few weeks after he went home, he died, although I never heard why.

The last of the comatose boys I cared for was Lenny, who was quite different from Sam or Jeff. I forget the cause of his trauma, but he was transferred to us from the ICU and was far more aware of his surroundings than Jeff had been. In bed, he sat up and looked around. In what the ICU staff must have thought was kindness, they'd taped his eyes open. That bothered me and was one detail I'd learned during my EMT training that applied to my hospital work.

One evening during the EMT classes, the physician who was teaching us showed a picture of a man with severely injured eyes. That was the result, he said, of a comatose victim after an ER left his eyes wide open for several hours. Not blinking, his eyes dried out. I worried that the same might happen to Lenny. So I played politics, bringing in one authority to counter another. I called the hospital's eye clinic, and they confirmed that his eyes should not be taped open. I told my nurse what I was doing and removed the tape. Not long afterward, he could keep his eyes open for himself, blinking when needed.

In fact over the next few days, his condition improved so rapidly, I reasoned that, if I were in his situation, I'd be dying for a bath. The nurse had gone to lunch, so I thought, "Why not ?" It would draw attention to him and show how rapidly he was getting better.

When my nurse came back, she asked, "Where's Lenny?" Comatose people don't get up and walk around, so I had a bit of fun casually telling her, "Oh, he's taking a bath." She was upset until I showed him in the tub, obviously loving it and easily able to keep his head above water.

Even better, his doctor came around to check up on him during the bath and, seeing that, made plans to transfer him to Rehab, where they could do much more for him than we could. He was transferred that very afternoon. Over the next few weeks I'd occasionally see him walking about with an attendant.

The great contrast between Sam, Jeff and Lenny illustrate that a diagnosis like "comatose" means little. It's a crude description rather than a specific diagnosis. People in comas are not necessarily 'brain dead' or in a 'vegetative state,' as some in the news media might like us to believe. Their conditions and awareness vary greatly, as does their future. If I'd been at the hospital longer, I could probably point to a recovery from even a severe coma. After all, when a light is turned off, we don't say the bulb is dead. We flip a switch and turn it on. In the future, we may discover how to turn on consciousness.

Finally, for several days I took care of Mimi, a fourteen-year-old girl whose initial diagnosis was a coma of unknown origin. From the start, however, she was thought to have catatonia, which the National Library of Medicine defines as: "A condition characterized by inactivity, decreased responsiveness to stimuli, and a tendency to maintain an immobile posture. The limbs tend to remain in whatever position they are placed (waxy flexibility)."

This might help you understand. On Hem-Onc, some of our children, having endured one round of chemotherapy, insisted on being drugged into oblivion for their later rounds. They were like rag dolls, floppy and not resisting any movement. In contrast, sleeping children are a little stiff when moved, having a position they unconsciously prefer. Those in comas are different yet again, often drawn up and strongly resisting stretching or bending.

Mimi was like none of those. The technical term is "waxy flexibility." Think the little bendable dolls that dancers use to illustrate dance moves and you'll understand. I turned her every couple of hours and, when I did, she offered only a little resistance. But once placed in a new position, however odd, she froze there, like wax that had cooled. To test what I'd been reading about catatonia, I lifted her arm up into the air and it remained there, only slowly sinking back to the bed. "Odd, really odd," I thought.

It took a couple of tries, but eventually our doctors confirmed Mimi's catatonia, broke her out of her unresponsiveness, and transferred her to the psychiatric ward of a nearby university hospital that was better equipped to handle her case. A friend who worked there as a psychiatric nurse told me that she stayed about three months before being released.

Next, we turn to one of the most moving experiences I had during my entire time at the hospital.

43. HANNA THE MOST BRAVE

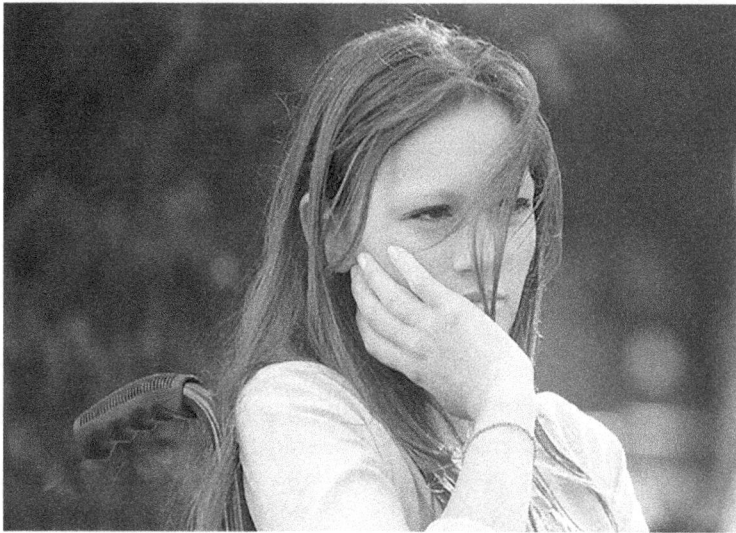

One nurse referred to the pair as "Mutt and Jeff," a humorous reference to an old newspaper comic strip about a friendship between two very different characters. She was right. These two girls were the most unlikely pair of friends you could imagine.

Tanya was tiny. I still have a picture of her. She was about twelve, but looked more immature than many nine-year-olds. She was also the quietest and most somber patient I ever had. Although I spoke with her often during the weeks I cared for her, I have trouble recalling anything she said in response. When you were with her, she would look at you silently with sad, soulful eyes.

Her opposite, Hanna, was about seventeen, large and chatty. She was also developmentally delayed, according to a psychological assessment, but with the confident, outgoing, highly sociable personality many such people have. That's what that nurse meant about Mutt and Jeff. These two girls could not have been more different.

Their medical situations also differed. Hanna was in for back surgery, but was otherwise healthy. She was up and about in her wheelchair, giving every appearance of robust good health. Tanya's situation was far grimmer. She had an inoperable brain tumor. Sadder still, for reasons that were never explained to us, no family member stayed with her during her final weeks. She'd been left all alone—abandoned.

As staff, we tried to see Hanna as often as possible, but, given our heavy workload, the friendship we could offer was limited. That's when the amazing happened. Tanya and Hanna—that most unlikely pair—became close friends, spending hours together, with Hanna talking and Tanya listening.

Keep in mind just how brave that was. Hanna knew she was choosing as a friend someone who would soon die, with all the pain that entailed. Even though we arranged with the Make a Wish Foundation for Tanya to have a trip to Disneyland, I am sure Hanna's freely given friendship must meant more to her than anything else in her brief life. We did what we could to help the two, arranging so they could spend as much time as possible together.

Finally, the day came. During the night, Tanya slipped into a coma. As I made my first rounds that morning, I looked in on her, making sure she seemed comfortable. She appeared relaxed and was breathing quietly, so I moved on. A short time later, the nurse came out of her room and told me she had died.

Sadly, with more time and better planning, we might have arranged for Hanna to be with her little friend to the very last. The usual start-of-shift rush prevented that. Now Hanna would have to be told. When I went into the room she shared with three other girls, she asked me how Tanya was doing. I didn't feel up to telling her myself, so I told her something that was technically true—that the last time I'd been in Tanya's room, she'd been sleeping quietly.

Then I went to the nurse. Knowing that she'd be much better than I at bearing the news, I told her that Hanna had asked about Tanya. She immediately went to Hanna, took her aside, and explained very lovingly what had happened. Then she took her into the room for one last visit with her sad, shy little friend.

We often imagine courage as something displayed by soldiers in battle or by fire fighters rushing into a burning building. But the courage that Hanna displayed when she chose to make the dying Tanya her special friend was the equal of any I've seen in my life.

44. AIR IN A CENTRAL LINE

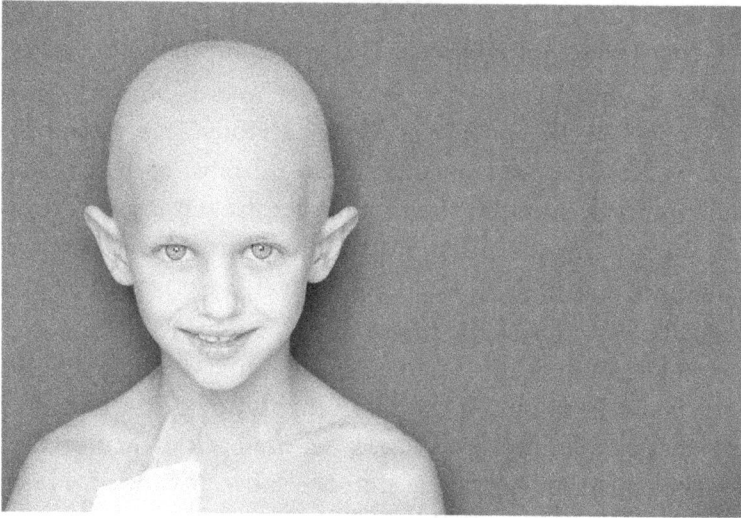

Early one sunny afternoon, I passed a room in which a girl of about fifteen was coughing. Hearing her, a thought flashed through my mind. A cough, particularly a shallow, rapidly repeated, tickle-in-the throat one, is one indication of an air embolism. I darted into her room, glanced at her central line, saw air rather than fluid, and moved quickly. As I asked her to turn on her left side, I switched off her IV pump with my right hand, and my left hand pulled the pillow out from under her head. I then elevated the foot of her bed. That would keep those evil air bubbles away from the left side of her heart and her brain, where they would do the most harm. When a physician arrived a few minutes later, all he added to what I'd already done was to have the girl breathe oxygen to more speedily clear the nitrogen from her blood.

Afterward, as I thought about what had happened, I realized I'd responded without asking myself, "What do I do next." My actions were one smooth motion without a wasted second. When you hear someone discuss an emergency situation during which their "training kicked in," that's what they're talking about. Properly trained and buttressed with experience, people know instinctively what to do. They don't panic. They don't flail about. They don't mutter to themselves. Most important of all, they don't look like a fool or hurt someone.

That's because good training frees you to think clearly. Years ago, when I climbed glaciated mountains, I practiced doing ice-axe arrests enough times that it became almost a reflex. A situation might arise when an arrest might save my life or someone else's. Fortunately, the only two times when I might have used the technique, it wasn't needed.

It was late afternoon. Another climber and I were coming down the rapidly darkening east side of Mount Rainier on a glacier that was steeper than I would have liked, with an unstable surface made up of few inches of loose snow on top of a harder, frozen layer. "We're going to slip," I warned myself. Still more troubling was an break in the glacier ahead that signaled an ice cliff. Tired as I was, I put myself on guard.

The guy below me was the first to lose his footing, yelling and tumbling down the slope. I knew the routine. I spun around and hurled myself at the snow, head uphill, the tip of my tightly gripped ice ax thrust as deeply as possible into the snow, with my back arched so the sharp crampon spikes on my boots dug into the snow. It worked. He was left suspended in the air below that ice cliff.

I might saved him from some dire fate, but I hadn't. The cliff was only about eight-feet high. The crevasse beneath if was only a few inches wide rather than a yawning pit hundreds of feet deep. He was uncomfortable, suspended in the air only by a waist strap, so he yelled for me to let him down, which I did. A minute later, it was my turn to slip, but knowing what he'd said, I didn't arrest myself. I slide happily over the cliff, plopping into the soft snow beyond.

That illustrates something important. As automatic as these trained responses can be, they don't make us robots. We can turn them off. By making complex actions a reflex, they free us to step back and ask ourselves, "Do I need to do this?" If we do, it's easy to trigger that reflex. In the case of an ice-axe arrest, I only needed to tell myself, "Arrest!" and the rest followed naturally. In the case of that girl, I needed only to think, "Air in line," to trigger the right response.

Many medical situations call for enough training, hands-on practice, and perhaps actual experience that what we do becomes that automatic. The bad news was that my response to that teen girl's air embolism wasn't the result of formal hospital preparation like my training in monitoring peritoneal dialysis had been. No class had taught me what to do. I was taught on the job by that first set of experienced nurses and that was backed up by sixteen months on Hem-Onc nights with those complex, error-prone, central-line IVs. What I did that afternoon was what I'd done several times before, getting quicker and more confident with each repetition. I'd learned by doing, and I'd learned well.

But then something occurred that bothered me. When I told the nurse I was working with that day what had happened, she looked shocked and told me that, if she'd been in my place, she would not have known what to do. And no, she wasn't a new nurse. What she'd confessed, while bad for our patients, wasn't her fault. She didn't know, because she had never been taught.

Some medical background will help you understand. You can see the dressing for a central line in the picture of The Girl at the start of this chapter. The line enters her chest below her right shoulder blade, runs just under her skin to make a longer path for any infection to travel, and then loops down to enter a large vein returning to her heart. Such lines are now common with cancer patients along with other systems called ports, which don't have an external line.

The particular central line we used had been invented by one of our doctors. Our hospital pioneered the routine use of it with pediatric cancer patients. That was good, but something else wasn't. The hospital had known for at least two years that it had a problem with a particular treatment combination: central venous lines, an IV pump with an unsafe, outdated design, and patients with complicated IVs. Each introduced risk. The combination was ticking time bomb.

On Hem-Onc, that combination was so common, we'd learned to cope. More experienced nurses taught newer nurses how to handle the problem. True, the system wasn't perfect. That informal mentoring system broke down when my first set of nurses left too quickly to train the second. But it did work, which is why I knew how to spot an embolism and respond in an instant. Unfortunately, that informal training wasn't good enough for the hospital as a whole. It taught *some* nurses *some* things they needed to know, but it didn't treat *every* nurse *everything* she needed to know.

I saw something similar one morning when I arrived on the teen unit to find a night nurse upset. She'd just discovered that she'd made a mistake with a teen-aged boy who had an inflammation of the bowels called Crohn's disease. To ease the burden on his digestive system, he'd been put on hyperalimentation (feeding by IV, also called Total Parenteral Nutrition or TPN). In his case, that meant two different IV fluids.

One was a brownish-yellow fluid that came in one-liter plastic IV bags. Because it contained almost all the nutrients we need in liquid form, it ran fast, often over a 100 cc an hour. The other came in small glass bottles and contained white, fat-like lipids and was given at a slower 10 to 15 cc an hour. The two could not have looked more different, but while setting his IV up in the dark, the nurse reversed the lines, running the lipids at the fast rate. She only discovered her mistake when the lipid bottle emptied just before seven, triggering an alarm.

Keep in mind that she wasn't inexperienced. In fact, I considered her one of the best young nurses in the hospital. She was the one who'd persuaded me to apply for the teen day shift. Yet she'd made an elementary mistake—one I touched on earlier. Most IV patients have uncomplicated IVs—one bag with one pump to give one medication every four hours. Those are easy to manage. When a patient's IV gets more complicated, a nurse has to consciously choose to be more careful. Doubling the complexity probably quadruples the chance of doing something wrong. Make any change at all, and she needed to step back and check everything—following every line from the bag through the pump to the patient. As carpenters say, "Measure twice, cut once." Doing otherwise courts disaster.

In the case of that boy with Crohn's, no harm was done. Lipids are not poison. He merely got in a couple of hours what he was supposed to get over an entire day. But in other situations, a mistake like that could be fatal. If that too-fast IV had been morphine, he'd have been dead.

Looking back, I wonder if hospitals might learn from the decks of aircraft carriers, where complex, dangerous operations have to be carried out under all weather conditions by deck crews who are often exhausted. If you watch a television documentary, you'll notice bright colored tags hanging beneath wings. Those tabs indicate a condition that must be changed before an aircraft takes off.

The hospital where I worked needed that. A nurse could be trained, before she made any changes to a patient's IV, to turn a tag around so a brightly colored side saying "Check IV" was visible. She wasn't to turn that tag back around to the dull-colored "IV OK" side until she'd consciously checked every item in the IV's flow. Flip the tag, make the change, check the IV, and then flip the tag back. It'd be an aid to memory, much like that pocket alarm I used to remind myself to check a child's temperatures in an hour.

That's not all. Checking IVs is straight-forward—just follow the fluid path. I could check even complicated, multi-pump IVs in a few seconds. But for more complicated situations, a checklist is better. Pilots use them during takeoffs and landings. Surgeons use them for operations. Nurses need checklists for complex procedures too.

Keep in mind that each of these aids to memory—reflexes, tags, and checklists—play different roles. Trained reflexes work best as responses to a clear and unambiguous stimulus, such as a heart monitor alarm triggering CPR. Tags remind us to do something, but don't give the specifics. Checklists tell us, step by step, what to do so nothing gets skipped. Each has its place.

To my great regret, at that time I wasn't thinking about how the nurses should be taught. I was focused on not making mistakes of my own. In that I was successful. During my two-plus years at the hospital, I worked over 4,000 hours, caring for hundreds of patients. I made tens of thousands of decisions without making a single mistake serious enough to become an incident report. I worked hard to achieve that.

That's good, but I should have done more. I should have also paid attention to how the system around me could be improved. Yes, I was being careful and learning from experience, but I wasn't sufficiently aware that either I and the nurses I worked with should be taught more, particularly in a formal, 'you must know this to work here' sense. In a hospital, *training before* a mistake is far better than bitterly *learning afterward*.

As I look back, what I regret most about the professional aspects of my time in the hospital was that I didn't draw attention to that failure to train. That's why I hope that this book will motivate those of you who go into medicine and nursing to look beyond just what you're doing. Don't be afraid to ruffle a few feathers in a good cause. Think constantly about what's happening around you and insist on good training. You might save someone's life and spare yourself years of hurt, bitterness and regret.

In the next chapter, we'll look at the unfortunate consequences of that failure to train, particularly when it involved common, well-known problems.

45. Conflict Spreads

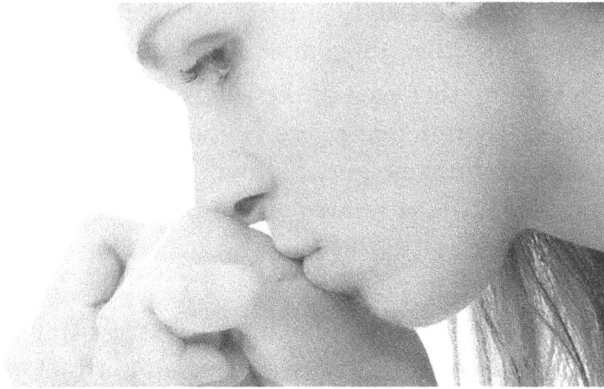

I had left Hem-Onc and the medical unit because I'd grown exhausted after 16 months on night shift, far longer than any nurse had worked before moving on. Even more important, I left because I felt frustrated, caught in a war between nurses that made it increasingly difficult to give our kids good care. One result has been a lifelong interest in work cultures and how they can be improved. That's one reason I wrote this book and why I hope you find it helpful.

At the time, I was confused about the cause of those clashes. At first, I placed the blame on a few ill-tempered nurses along with the poor people skills of a particular head nurse. Unhappy with their own lives and not inclined to be kind, they made everyone around them miserable. The result was a blame culture. Nurses felt they could only protect themselves by attacking others. Growing tensions, low morale, and more mistakes were the inevitable result. The feeble attempts I made to turn things around got nowhere.

In retrospect, I should have used the credibility I'd worked hard to build. I could have scheduled an appointment with the hospital's nursing administrator and shared my concerns. Unfortunately, at that time I was too exhausted to think about the larger picture. I wanted relief, so I transferred to the teen unit, which I knew was free of conflict.

That held true for about six months of the ten months I worked there. The key reason, I realized later, was that a nurse was filling in for the head nurse, who was on maternity leave. She was remarkably sweet and easy-going, with no ambition to move into administration. She was only serving in the role because someone had to do it. Although I didn't realize it at the time, her disinterest in an administrative career was shielding us.

Then the head nurse returned, and I soon sensed trouble. This time, it wasn't tension between nurses. On day shift, those relationships were too good to immediately turn sour. Instead, I saw a top-down attempt to stir up fear and conflict. We were expected to become informers, protecting ourselves by criticizing others. What had happened on the medical unit had seemed clumsy and accidental. This was deliberate.

In conversations with the returning head nurse, I was told that the hospital would be changing its staffing policies, reducing the number of aide positions like mine. That made no sense, I thought. Aides were so busy doing work for which we were well qualified, we hardly got a moment's rest. It made no sense to pay nurses, who made more money, to do simple things such as pass out food trays. Looking back, I suspect her claims were bogus, meant only to generate fear. Since I was planning to leave, she got nowhere. Besides, I don't scare easily.

The head nurse was also telling everyone that nursing on the unit was badly done and that she intended to set things right. There were crude hints that some nurses would go if they didn't change. That was nonsense. These were good nurses who were working almost unbelievably hard. I've already shared my belief that more formal, incident-based training for nurses was needed. That was true. But it was also true that there wasn't a nurse on the unit who wasn't highly motivated. On day shift, they were doing good work despite being dreadfully overworked. It was grossly unfair to beat up on them.

Soon, I was seeing the head nurse making the same clumsy attempts to manufacture mistakes that'd irked me on the medical unit. In my case, unable to come up with an actual incident against me—there were none—the head nurse poured over the flow sheets for who knows how long and discovered what she thought was a serious omission on my part. Get ready to be shocked by what she regarded as my gross incompetence. On the medical unit, I'd been attacked for putting something real and important into the flow sheets—a girl dying without family or visitors. This time I'd be attacked for not writing down something unnecessary.

An strong, athletic boy of about seventeen had been in for a brief course of that "chemotherapy drug-from-hell called cisplatin" that I mentioned earlier. Given my hatred for the drug, I remembered him well. I also remember taking care to notice what matters most with cisplatin—that he made those two-hour voids. Day shift made getting them easier. His IV rate, I also remember, was quite high, over 200 cc/hour. That's almost five liters or well over a gallon a day. If it hadn't been high, rest assured, I'd have squawked. I hated that drug.

Yet my head nurse seem to regard my care of that boy as a dismal failure. Did anything happen to him? No. Did I fail to get any of those necessary voids? No, my care of him was textbook perfect.

Grasping at straws, she was faulting me for not noting in the flow sheets that his voiding was sufficient. "That makes no sense," I thought. Flow sheets are for recording numbers, particularly the flow of fluids such as IVs and urine. They're not intended for detailed commentary on a patient's care, and aren't designed for that. Besides, it was silly to clutter flow sheets with what wasn't happening. We don't record "Patient did not die this shift' remarks." She was engaged in a witch hunt, and I wasn't the only victim. Virtually everyone was getting attacked in much the same way. Day nurses had it much worse than I.

As on the medical unit, perhaps I should have taken my complaint over her head. But by that point, I was planning to leave. I'd been accepted into a graduate program in medical ethics at the University of Washington's Medical School. Spring classes were approaching. I had savings, so I didn't need to stay at what was rapidly becoming an unpleasant place to work.

The head nurse also wanted me to find fault with nurses. That I refused to do. In fact, when I resigned I did the opposite. I gave the nurses I was working with a parting gift. I suspected our head nurse was trying to impress her superiors by claiming that things had gone badly while she was away, and that she was cracking the whip to restore discipline. That was not only utter bosh, it was a major blunder. In her efforts to impress her superiors, she hadn't noticed changes that really did need to be made. Her bureaucratic game—and a game it was—had been poorly thought out. That left her vulnerable.

So when I turned in my letter of resignation, I offered three suggestions to improve conditions for the day staff. It's been a long time, and I've forgotten the specifics, but I remember my intent well.

Day shift, I told the hospital's highest ranking nurse, was greatly overworked, while evening shift, with the same staffing level, had it easy. I knew that for a fact, since I'd dropped by in the evening. On one occasion, I found a nurse in a patient's bed watching television.

The solution was simple. Every responsibility that could be moved from day to evening should be moved. For nurses, that included the pre-surgery paperwork. Day nurses often found themselves having to do that just minutes before a teen was due to leave. Evenings could easily do it.

For aides that included showers and baths. Both were a disaster on days. Send a teen off for a shower, and soon afterward a doctor or lab technician might show up needing to see him or her. That made no sense, I told her. Evenings were best, and evenings had the time.

Needless to say, the head nurse was not happy when I met with her one last time. My letter had apparently looked—as intended—as a recital of the reasons I was leaving, even though the primary reason was my return to school. Since I had a good reputation, the head of nursing had called her in wanting answers.

In responding, the head nurse denied that any of the problems I described existed. Since she'd not raised them, she had to do that to play her bureaucratic game. But she was wrong. Although I hadn't told anyone on staff about those three needed changes, two were so obvious they came up at a staff meeting a few days after my letter—perhaps stimulated by rumors about my letter. Denying that too-heavy day workload was the head nurse's big mistake. She'd have been wiser to observe what was actually happening before she beginning her attacks. But only good managers look before they leap. They're also careful with criticism.

Next we look at later events. As aware as I was at what was happening when I left, even I was surprised with what followed.

46. Nurses Flee

About three months after I quit working at the hospital, I attended a town meeting at a local television station. I've forgotten the topic, but recall it had something to do with medicine.

The hospital's chaplain was also there, saw me, and sat down next to me. Imagine Mr. Rogers of the television reruns, and you'll grasp his personality. A most gentle and kind man, he was troubled by what was happening at the hospital and wanted my insights.

From him, I discovered that I'd left just before a flood of nurse resignations. A nurse had been quiting almost every week day. Staffing on the hospital's floors was now some 40 nurses (or 20 percent) below the minimum necessary to run the hospital and hiring new nurses had become almost impossible.

The last fact I already knew. Then in the early stages of graduate studies, I was taking undergrad classes with nursing students and back-to-school nurses. When I mentioned where I'd worked, their response was invariably, "That terrible place, I'd never work there." The trouble I'd seen was now common knowledge in the nursing community.

I also knew why those nurses were leaving. Morale on the medical unit had been bad for over a year. That's why I'd transferred. Morale on the teen unit was turning sour when I resigned. Apparently, I'd just beat some of its nurses out the door.

It gets worse. According to the chaplain, to get enough staffing, the hospital was requiring nurses to work overtime well in excess of the maximum allowed by their contract. I knew what that meant—endless twelve-hour shifts. Work repeated twelve-hour days with few days off and your job becomes your life. Add in the time it takes to sleep, eat, shower, dress and commute, and you have almost no free time.

Nurses at the hospital fell into two broad groups. Each would respond differently. The largest group were those who placed their first priority on kids and were a joy to work with. I suspect some of them were among the first to leave, frustrated as I had been by their inability to halt the downward slide. Those who remained once the staffing numbers plummeted were the unfortunate ones. Their strong sense of responsibility would keep them there to make sure kids still got good care. "Don't punish these kids for problems that aren't of their doing," would be their attitude. That's why staffing hadn't sunk even lower.

A smaller group were those I called 'Witch Nah' nurses, my own poor pun for the name of the state nurse union. From the start, I had mixed feelings about the union. On one hand, it was obvious that nurses are often so badly put upon by hospitals, they need a powerful, united voice. That was particularly true where I was working because, as one nurse told me, the hospital's administration felt it had nurses in a bind. If they wanted to work in pediatrics, they had little choice but to work there. Compounding the problem, she said, was that nurses at a children's hospital could not win a dispute by threatening to strike. The public would never look with favor on such a strike, and many nurses would refuse join it.

On the other hand, the nurse union often seemed focused on the interests of politicized and less talented nurses at the expense of all nurses, much less of patients. Those who are good at what they do are hard to replace and there's significant power in that. In contrast, those who lack talent also lack job security. Firing them will almost inevitably mean a more qualified replacement. They are the ones who love union rules and contracts. My prejudice—if that's what it was—had been increased by the fact that those ill-tempered 'rhymes with witches' nurses were active in the union. Unions and enjoying your work rarely mix.

That said, at that time the union certainly had issues that mattered, particularly the climate of harsh, unfair criticism and the contractual working-hour violations. The same formal grievance process that makes it hard to fire incompetent nurses also protects talented nurses who're being unfairly treated. In fact, during my last months at the hospital, I was surprised to discover that I was beginning to feel that the union had a useful role. Before that, I'd considered them irrelevant. I suspect nurses who'd been indifferent to the union were going through that same change of mind. Better flawed protection than no protection.

Yes, it was probably true that the union was doing little constructive as matters turned sour. That makes sense. Unions often *want* their members to have bad relationships with management, since that enhances a union's power. When all is well, nurses feel more allegiance to their employer, who pays them, than to a distant, dues-grabbing union. Bad management and bad unions may even find themselves in a perversely symbiotic relationship. Each needs the other to maintain a tense and unhealthy status quo.

I just checked that union's website. Emblazoned across their home page alongside a picture of a tired nurse in surgical scrubs, is news that a bill "limiting mandatory overtime" had just passed the state house of representatives. Obviously, the problems that haunted the hospital then, particularly inadequate staffing corrected by excess overtime, still exist. For a number of reasons, the website said, present-day hospitals have too-few nurses and have been using various tricks, such as "pre-scheduled on-call" to fill gaps. The union's argument makes sense. Tired nurses do have trouble giving good care. I experienced that myself. It's also true that having too few nurses on duty is dangerous. Treating the sick isn't like repairing a car. If a hospital lacks enough staff for the work load, it can't simply park sick people on some back lot until later.

Returning to that televised town meeting, the hospital's chaplain asked me why I thought nursing there was in such turmoil. At the time I didn't have a good answer. About a year earlier, I'd lain the blame for the trouble in the medical unit on its most obvious cause, several ill-tempered day nurses aided and abetted by a head nurse who knew little about managing people. As the teen unit began its downward spiral, however, I could see that the troubles weren't coming from the nurses. Day shift wasn't cursed with a single, ill-tempered nurse, perhaps because only young and energetic nurses could keep up the brutal pace. No, there the only visible cause was that just-returned head nurse. She was finding faults where none existed and blind to the real issues.

Were a few bad apples among the hospital's head nurses the cause of the troubles? When I'd left, that made sense. It explained why, despite a grueling workload, morale was good on the teen unit until the head nurse returned. But what I heard from nurses in class suggested that wasn't the whole story. Not counting specialty clinics, there were about seven to nine nursing units in the hospital. Each had someone in a head nurse role. A hospital isn't a barrel of fruit. Two bad apples would not make the entire barrel rotten and certainly not that quickly. Remember too that the nurses I met on campus weren't talking about not working on specific units. They were warning not to work at the hospital at all.

Blaming a few bad head nurses also made little sense from what I had seen when I floated to other units. In my experience, the head nurses fell into three roughly equal groups.

Where I floated the most, the unit for babies under one, always struck me as well-led, with good morale and confident, happy, baby-loving nurses. That, I thought with envy, must come from having a gifted head nurse, one who knew nursing, cared about her nurses and helped them give good care.

Other head nurses were in the middle. They were like the temporary nurse on teens. She wasn't a talented administrator, because she didn't want to be one. These head nurses did their job well enough not to create new problems, but they didn't solve existing ones, such as the overwork on the teen day shift.

It was the third group that drew my attention. To my untutored eye, they were grossly unqualified. Being a head nurse is more than filling out a work roster each week. A head nurse lies at the intersection between management and nurses. Management sees through the eyes of head nurses and it speaks to nurses though them. They play a critical role in staff morale. When they behave badly, morale plummets.

A good head nurse, I thought, needs to be first and foremost a good nurse. But even as an aide with little formal training, I saw that often wasn't true. Bad nurses seemed drawn into administration. Partly, that was to escape a job they did poorly. Partly it was because some clearly disliked caring for patients. Unfortunately, a nurse who dislikes patients becomes a head nurse who dislikes nurses. That was bad, bad, bad.

In contrast, the gifted nurses I met typically moved into more specialized areas that used their talents and kept them in close contact with patients. Looking back, I wonder why hospitals in general weren't making head nurse positions more attractive to those nurses. A nurse who enjoys giving good care to a dozen patients might enjoy helping a dozen nurses offer good care to many dozens of patients.

Something else was not right. Why did moving into administration mean losing touch with patients? That draws bad nurses into administration and repels good ones. And why isn't a head nurse considered a mentor, circulating among her nurses like a nurse does among her patients, learning first hand about problems and helping out? Most paperwork and staffing assignments could be handled by a clerk.

On nights, I'd tried excuse the head nurse. She wasn't around when we were working, I told myself. She got her wrong ideas from those dreadful 'rhymes with witches' day nurses. That sort of thing. But working days, I realized that wasn't the entire story. On teens, I rarely saw the head nurse, even though her office was just yards away. On both units, there simply wasn't that much contact between the head nurse and nursing staff. That's why she saw failures where there were none, and why she didn't grasp just how overworked our day nurses were or how poor their formal, on-the-job training had become.

That could have been different. The hospital desperately needed head nurses who circulated constantly among their staff, and who came in early or stayed late to have contact with other shifts. It needed nurses who were sympathetic to nursing concerns, less likely to be critical, and talented enough to take on much of the training themselves. And yes, that meant doing things differently. That's precisely my point. Since the hospital's problems flowed from excessive criticism, a more sympathetic head nurse, one willing to take up the cause of nurses, would have been a major plus. Low morale and high turnover are expensive and result in costly mistakes. If that meant paying head nurses more to lure them away from specialty nursing, it would be money well spent.

Of course, I also came to realize that the problem must run deeper than just bad head nurses. More was involved. Why, I asked myself, would a hospital choose to hire unqualified head nurses in the first place? That made no sense. Why did it have policies that discouraged talented nurses from becoming head nurses? The specialty nurses I knew loved to teach. Also, why were head nurses placed in an adversarial relationship with nurses and isolated from those they supervised? Finally, how could a situation like this grow so bad that nurses fled and care at the entire hospital suffered? We take that up next.

47. Larger Issues

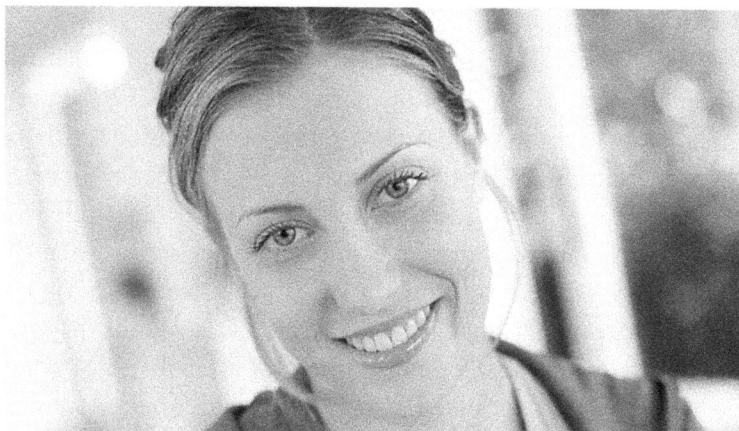

The summer after I left the hospital, I decided to make my vacation a drive up to Canada to attend a medical ethics conference at the University of British Columbia. There I met a nursing professor who answered a question that had troubled me for months.

"Why do hospitals employ head nurses who're obviously incompetent?," I asked her. To me, that made no sense. No auto repair shop would knowingly hire a shop supervisor who didn't understand cars. Why hire someone who was, at best, a mediocre nurse, as well as a dreadful manager? A bad nurse could not teach good nursing. A bad manager could not motivate nurses. I'd seen that happen twice, and it seemed crazy.

The nursing professor knew precisely what I meant. Quick as a flash, she responded, "Because they want someone who'll do what they say." Compliance trumps competence. Was it really that simple?

I want to be fair. Step back and look at what administrators face. Not all changes are popular. Some trigger resistance. A head nurse secure in her abilities may protest or simply ignore policies she feels are foolish. One that's less capable is more compliant, particularly if she fears not finding another job. She does as she is told, perhaps even with an excess of zeal. Lacking good sense about people, hierarchy is all she understands. She'll pander to those over her and bully those under her.

That's what I'd seen, particularly the attacks on skilled and hard-working young nurses. A failure herself, this sort of head nurse would see other nurses either as failure-prone or as threats to her due to their talent. Making mistakes herself, she sees other nurses as mistake prone. Fearing criticism, she creates a climate of fear. Not good at teaching or learning, she doesn't value training.

Years later I gained further insight when I read an article on management roles. The lowest level of management, it said, has a stressful but critical role. It's where those who make policies interact those who do things. In a hospital that role is filled by head nurses. Above are administrators. Below are nurses. To work effectively, the article went on, the lowest level, must be a shock absorber. Policies come down that are poorly worded, ill-timed, or even stupid. It's the role of the lowest-level manager to contest that change or, if that's likely to fail, to ignore it. "Our workers are lazy. Push them harder," is a terrible idea when employees are overworked, stressed out, and expected to do more than humanly possible—day shift on the teen unit.

For a talented supervisor, noncompliance with folly makes good sense. In the case of a hospital, if she carries out bad orders, her most capable, experienced nurses will leave. They're the ones who have the best chances of finding other jobs quickly. They may be replaced by less experienced, less motivated nurses. That means trouble.

I wasn't a fly on a wall in the administration, so I don't know what was happening outside the two units where I worked. But I suspect the work climate that had nurses fleeing and other nurses refusing to apply had to come from the top down. That's probably the only way the troubles could have become so pervasive. Perhaps the problem ended at the nursing administration. More likely, it went higher still.

Highest of all was the hospital's chief administrator, because he was where all responsibilities stopped. He and I met exactly twice, and both were revealing. The first came when I was hurrying to an 8 a.m. CPR instructors meeting in one of the small meeting rooms next to the cafeteria. I'd worked all night, I was tired, and I wanted to get the meeting over so I could sleep. When you work nights, sleep becomes an obsession. I also felt that the little overtime I earned teaching CPR classes wasn't worth the disruption in my sleep schedule. I only taught out of a sense of duty. Someone had to do it.

Arriving a few minutes early, I barged into a meeting he was hosting. He was obviously ticked off at my interruption, but I didn't care and didn't hide that. Our meeting and time were posted by the door. By the

My Nights with Leukemia

rules, he should have already vacated the room. As I recall, I even reminded him that the room was now ours.

He and I met again in a hallway one morning a few weeks later, and I could tell he recognized me. I found it intriguing that he smiled and seemed genuinely friendly. My conclusion at the time still seems true. He was an expert in the push and shove of administrative politics. Anyone in his position would have to be. He'd taken my measure and concluded that, despite my lowly position, I was someone who wouldn't be intimidated. That meant I had to be dealt with, at least on the personal level, as an equal. To his credit, he seemed willing to do that.

That's why I think much of what I'll be describing next was unnecessary. Some leaders are narcissistic autocrats, unwilling to admit they can be wrong. I don't think that was true in this case. From my brief encounters with both the hospital's director and the head of nursing, they seemed capable, responsible people. The ultimate fault, I believe, did not lie with them. It lay with their response to major changes taking place in medicine at the time.

Shortly after I left the hospital, I studied those changes in graduate school. This was a time where broad, national changes in hospital care were creating disruptions whose consequences no one understood.

The first was a new idea being pushed onto hospitals by the federal government called diagnostic-related groups or DRGs. Traditionally, hospital medicine had been based on a fee-for-service model linked directly to the treatment given. In our hospital, at the foot of every child's bed was a sheet of paper with a name and patient number. When we started an IV, for instance, each item we used came with a yellow label that was to be placed on that sheet. Similar charges were made for drugs and lab tests. Most services meant more fees and thus more income.

That meant that the more a hospital did, the more it could charge. Critics claimed that encouraged hospitals to over-treat and keep patients hospitalized longer than necessary. Their solution was the DRG. When a patient entered the hospital, he or she would be assigned to one of thousands of DRGs, depending on their diagnosis and the severity of their illness. What the hospital was paid was determined by that DRG. Treat cheaply, quickly and efficiently, and the hospital might turn a little profit. Treat less efficiently, and the hospital lost money. Given how unpredictable a disease can be, it's easy to see why DRGs had hospital administrators worried. Also, keep in mind that most of those I worked with were kind and capable people. Their treatments weren't driven by finances. A new IV—with all the accompanying pain and trauma for a child—would only be started because it was necessary for the child and not to run up a bill.

The other change pushed hospitals in the opposite direction and was the result an explosion in malpractice settlements. In the past, ambulance-chasing lawyers had focused on those who'd caused an injury, for instance, suing trucking firms or automobile insurance companies for huge sums. Growth in that area was limited, so these anything-for-a-buck lawyers were focusing on what happened to a patient after he reached the hospital. Not only did hospitals have 'deeper pockets'—meaning more money—than the general public, hospitals offered numerous opportunities to sue. Hospital staff make many decisions and it only takes one wrong deed—or one right one that can be made to look wrong—to provide grounds for a huge lawsuit. Worse still, I've had enough experience with lawyers to know that some are quite willing to do almost anything, including twist facts and lie, to get money. Even practicing good medicine isn't enough to protect a hospital or a doctor from a lying and manipulative lawyer.

The result was an explosion in malpractice claims and payments. A few years after I left the hospital, I took a community college class taught by lawyers. In one class the lawyer-instructor attempted to make malpractice lawyers look less greedy by pointing out just how rapidly the revenues of insurance companies had risen. I felt like shouting, "Liar," because on the same screen (but unmentioned by him) was a chart of the payments those insurance companies were paying out. Insurance company income had risen six-fold because the payments they were making had also risen six-fold in just a few years. The insurance companies weren't doing any better. It was the tort lawyers who were making out like bandits, typically taking a third of those huge settlements.

Now imagine yourself a hospital administrator trapped in that new and growing horror of horrors. On one hand, your income is likely to be reduced in unpredictable ways by DRGs. On the other hand, your insurance costs are being driven upward, rapidly and equally unpredictably, by malpractice claims. The only way you know to respond to the first is to reduce costs. The only way you know how to respond to the second is to practice expensive defensive medicine—over-testing and over-treating so you look good in court. The clash inherent in those two contrary pressures generates fear. In our case, that fear was transferred onto the most readily available target—the nurses—in the wrong-headed belief that pressure would make them *less* rather than *more* prone to make mistakes.

That fits with what I suspected at the time—that there'd been some costly lawsuits involving nursing errors. It'd be easy for an administrator to assume those lawsuits were the result of increasingly poor nursing rather than increasingly aggressive lawyers. And while nurses were saying that work stress going up due to a more difficult patient load, I suspect that much of that stress was a result of fear-inducing hospital policies and less emphasis on appropriate training.

Keep in mind that the hospital's decision to apply pressure on nurses wasn't that unusual. When I was majoring in engineering, we were warned that, "When you're up to your neck in alligators, it's hard to remember that your original goal was to drain the swamp." Trapped between federal DRGs and the greedy lawyers, the hospital seems to have forgotten that its real purpose was to treat sick children. Unable to shape national trends, it focused on the most readily available target. In most hospitals, unfortunately, that's the nurses. That's hardly surprising. Those in charge—administrators and doctors—have a vested interest in shifting the blame off themselves.

In the short-term, the hospital responded badly. In the long-term, it seems to have learned from its mistakes. When I was there, the hospital hired nurses just out of school, intending teach them what they needed to know. When it failed to put enough emphasis on teaching, relying instead in threats, all the troubles I've described naturally followed.

Today, nurses who work there tell me that, in general, a nurse must get her training elsewhere, so mostly experienced nurses are hired. Also, judged by what the hospital has posted on line, there's a much greater stress on on-the-job training. That's good. Training shouldn't be allowed to just happen. It needs to be aggressive, anticipating problems and constantly evaluated for effectiveness. There must to be staff for whom training is their prime responsibility. Head nurses and nurses also need to be encouraged to make suggestions and new technology should be used to make that training better. And head nurses should be, first and foremost, talented nurses and gifted teachers.

48. WINNING A SMILE

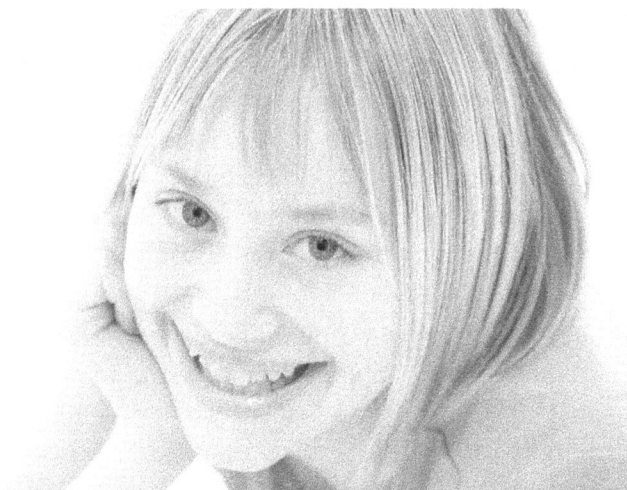

Now for something that's far more uplifting than accounts of long-ago squabbling and its unfortunate results. The best counter to a life in medicine or nursing that's built around either the ability to endure a grind or one built on an addiction to excitement is one established on life-affirming reasons. There's a video on YouTube that illustrates that perfectly.

The homemade video opens with the words, "Once upon a time... there lived a little princess in a place called Brazil. She had a friend she hid behind." That friend proves to be a fuzzy, bright-pink doll with a large and most-symmetric smile. We soon discover the reason this little girl hides behind her doll's face. Her own face is marred by a cleft lip.

The captioning continues, "along came a team of funny people... Operation Smile. With a funny camera you could see yourself in." The little girl waves at the camera and smiles her lopsided little smile.

Then it's the next day and the "funny people" return with their "funny camera." We see her cleft lip has been surgically corrected, although she's apparently not yet seen the results. Looking ever so serious, she waves for that funny camera again. A caption now reads, "Camera screen flips over. Her eyes will tell you when."

They're right. We can easily tell when she sees the new her. Her beautiful, dark Latin eyes light up, and she stares intensely at the screen. Then her surgeon, still in his green scrubs, crouches beside her and encourages her to move toward the camera. She studies closely her new face. As she does, her mouth opens wide and, turning to her surgeon, she makes a gesture like she's feeding herself. Eating must have been difficult with that cleft lip.

She turns back to the camera, experiments with her new smile, and begins to wave enthusiastically, a huge smile lighting up her face. The camera zooms back and a Brazilian nurse joins the two in waving at the camera. At the end, with the nurse's encouragement, the little girl blows a kiss at the camera.

In medicine and nursing, as in any profession, it's easy to get so caught up in what we are doing—meaning the techniques and skills that a job requires—that we forget what that amateur video demonstrates perfectly, the why behind the what. The first time I saw that video I thought, "If anything would get me to endure the long, grueling process to become a pediatric surgeon, that video would be it."

Without the right motivations, our ability to endure the inevitable drudgery, discouragement, and defeat fades. With it, over time even the adrenaline-pumping excitement of an ER or ICU dims. In my case, when you're surrounded by dreadfully sick and often dying children, it's all to easy to forget why you are there and get depressed. In the case of administrators, it was the seeming impossibility of fighting distant bureaucrats and grasping lawyers.

How did I fight it? Grinds demoralize. I didn't want my work to become a grind and I certainly didn't want to become a slacker, doing only what was demanded. Each evening as I arrived at work, I reminded myself just what was happening around me. I promised that I'd do all I could to give these children the greatest possible chance at life or, failing that, the best possible death. What happened to me, I told myself, mattered little. What happened to them mattered a lot.

I kept in mind that working on Hem-Onc made it was "easy to be good." By that I didn't mean the work itself was easy. The demands were high, the stress was great, and the nights seemed endless. No, it was easy because the choices I faced were stark. I knew precisely what I should do. Good and right were clear.

Yes, some nights I could have said to myself: "It is the middle of the night and I'm bone tired. I've had only four hours sleep in the last twenty-four. My skin feels prickly and my eyes burn. These kids are stable.

There's no reason to keep constantly circulating and checking on them. Slow down and relax. Nothing will happen tonight."

But I knew that was a lie. Our kids were always mere inches away from disaster. There was always the possibility that a child would suffer or die because of me. When I put it in terms that blunt, it was "easy to be good." My motivation lay in constantly reminding myself how important what I did was. The little speed bumps in my personal life mattered little in comparison to the towering mountains and plunging cliffs these children faced. I wasn't going to die. They might.

That's true in much of what we do. Viewed rightly, even the most mundane-seeming jobs can be life-changing. If as a guy I were to rate jobs that "don't matter much," I'd be tempted to include working in a beauty salon. After all, adding highlights to a woman's hair doesn't quite rank with correcting a little girl's cleft palate or preventing a boy from dying of leukemia.

But that's not completely true. To support my writing, I sometimes did inside security at private events. A few years ago I worked at a Christmas party for the employees of a small beauty salon chain. I was surprise to discover that the salon's two owners weren't talking about profits and wages, which is what most businesses talk about at such events. No, they were encouraging their employees to describe situations where their work had made a difference in lives.

The one I remember best involved a woman who came in for a 'makeover' just before her wedding. The beautician encouraged her to go for broke, including dying her hair a lovely blonde. The woman left delighted by her new look. Two days later, that beautician got a call from the woman's mother. The mother wanted to thank her for what she'd done. Her daughter, it seemed, had been about to marry a jerk, but was so delighted by her much-improved appearance, she gained enough confidence to call the wedding off. She'd wait for someone better.

An even more telling experience came when someone who worked for a community college asked me to mail old textbooks that taught keyboard skills to Bangladesh for a small, New Zealand-based relief organization. She'd gotten her college to donate those textbooks, but needed someone to handle the international shipping.

That proved easy enough. I mailed the books and thought no more about it until I heard the globe-trotting president of that organization mention that in most countries he visited, it took weeks to get a visa to the next country he was to visit. Bangladesh, he said, was an incredible exception. There, his visa often came back approved in two days.

Why? Grasp what his organization did there and you'll understand. Those textbooks I'd sent were for a school it ran in the nation's capital. It taught English and office skills to young women who had been forced into the city by the poverty of their rural families. With their new skills, those women got good jobs. Some were working for embassies.

Thinking about that, I realized something remarkable was happening. With no marketable skills, when those young women first arrived in capitol, they were often forced toward prostitution. The school meant the difference between one of the worst jobs and one of the best.

Now imagine that president's visa request arriving at an embassy. The person handling incoming mail recognizes the organization, and knows a secretary who went to the school. Bypassing the usual laggardly procedures, he gives it to that secretary. The secretary knows how to speed up a visa approval. Although she has a lot to do, for her there's nothing more important than this. If a stamped approval is needed, she goes to the person who has that stamp. If a signature is required, even if it's the signature of the ambassador himself, she gets it, perhaps with the help of another graduate. As a result, a visa application that came in the morning mail might go out in the afternoon mail.

Does all that go against the embassy's established policies? Almost certainly. Does it put this secretary at risk of being criticized by the more bureaucratic-minded? It does, much as my own efforts to right a wrong led me to clash with head nurses. But that secretary has motivations that go beyond the mundane. In her case, that's showing appreciation. A Brazilian child with a beautiful new smile and a visa returned in the same day it demonstrate that something good has been done. That's what makes any job meaningful.

Doing something because it is good for others is the foundation on which all good medical and nursing care should be built. It's where everyone from minor hospital staff (such as me) to the most senior physicians and administrators should be looking for inspiration. It's where they can find the strength to fight the unhealthy pressures of a hospital floor and destructive changes in national health practices. With those words I close this book. A sample chapter from the companion volume follows.

49. Much-loved Binky

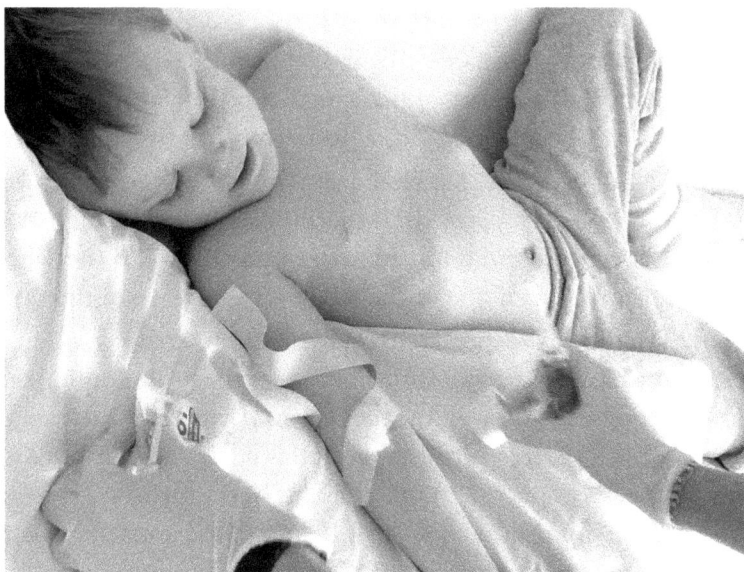

This chapter comes from the companion volume, *Hospital Gowns and Other Embarrassments*. That book builds on my experience working on the hospital's busy adolescent unit. It's a practical how-to guide for patients, telling them how to manage situations they may find embarrassing and make their stay more enjoyable. While its primary audience is teen girls, the advice is helpful for anyone facing hospitalization.

The first time I went to Binky's bed, I saw a homemade sign at the foot saying, "I know I'm special because God don't make no junk." Whoever made the sign, his mother or a nurse, was right. He was a most special little boy.

Binky was about four years old. With spindly limbs and a swollen belly, he looked like the Kermit the Frog doll that someone had left in his bed. He had Prune Belly Syndrome, which meant his belly was a mess. The name comes from the fact that, born without abdominal muscles, the belly of a baby with the syndrome can be as wrinkled as a dried prune. Binky was also missing some organs. He had only one kidney and no bladder. His diaper needed to be placed near his belly button, because that was where the urine dribbled out, one drop at a time.

Yet despite all the added work Binky created, he was an absolute joy to care for. Just coming up to his bed would make me feel better. I still remember one day when the order came to remove the NG (nasogastric, meaning nose-to-stomach) tube we'd been using to feed him formula. The tube is soft and doesn't hurt when in place. But going down and coming up, it creates a choking sensation as the tip passes through the lower throat. I was trying to be careful with that when he expressed concern for me. In spite of all he was going through, he was more worried about my feelings than his own. That was Binky, a most incredible kid.

As you might expect, the nursing staff doted on this wonderful little guy and, given the severity of his sickness, quite a few staff throughout the hospital got to know him. His dying was a long, downward spiral. His one kidney began to fail, dialysis was impossible for anyone as frail as he, and every effort to adjust his diet came to naught. The night he died, one of the evening aides—on her own initiative—stayed to be with him, holding his hand until his family arrived.

After his death, his family, knowing how special he was to staff, held a memorial service just for us. They knew our shifts and picked the best possible time, which was in early afternoon. But that only meant that attending was equally difficult for everyone. For those on nights like me it meant getting up at what our bodies thought was three a.m. For those on days, it meant finding someone willing to come in early to cover for them. For those on evenings, it meant finding someone on days who'd stay over until they could get to work. The result was a lot of people making a special effort to honor one little boy. No less that twenty-four nurses and aides came to honor Binky.

Why were so many people willing to give something extra to care for Binky while he was alive and to make a special effort to honor him after he was dead? Sick and frail, Binky had nothing of material value to give us. It was the little things he did all the time, particularly the appreciation he showed for what we did for him. When I did something, he'd thank me, even when he was so weak, he could barely gasp out the words. You cared about him because he cared about you.

Why did that create such strong bonds? Because, as strange as it sounds, expressing gratitude and concern for caregivers are rare in hospitals. Does that mean our patients didn't appreciate what we were doing? Not at all. I had kids who liked me. The mother of a little girl from

Hem-Onc brought her by to see me on the teen unit after my transfer. As soon as the girl saw me, she threw herself out of her mother's arms and into mine. She was delighted to see the guy who'd sung her to sleep, night after night, with off-key renditions of "You are my sunshine."

No, the problem wasn't a lack of appreciation. It was that these kids, from babies to teens, often faced problems so overwhelming it was difficult for them to take their eyes off their own fears and suffering. We were strong, we were healthy, and we seemed emotionally together. What need did we have? And yet we did, as the response to Binky reveals. We needed to their thanks and appreciation.

That's the magic tip I'm offering you. When you're in a hospital and feeling overwhelmed, take a moment to say something kind to those caring for you. Thank them even for little things. If a nurse reaches over and adjusts your pillow, show your appreciation. If you're so sick you can barely gasp out the words, the nurse will be even more impressed. If those caring for you seemed stressed out—as they usually are—say something like, "I can tell you're busy today. Thanks for helping me."

Remember, you're stuck in that bed with nothing else to do. You might as well be kind and thoughtful. It certainly beats being crabby and critical. Look for ways to compliment staff. If the hospital allows a nurse to dress distinctively, find something to praise about her outfit. When I worked with little kids, I clipped a little Kola bear to my stethoscope to make it more friendly. If you see something like that, mention it. Take the time to see them as people. Learn their names and something about them. Remember their days off and mention missing them when they come back. If a nurse said something about going for a hike, ask her how it went. She's caring for you. Show you care about her.

Don't forget humor, which works wonders in tense situations. Look on the Internet for stories about how President Ronald Reagan responded after almost being killed by an assassin. As a patient, he impressed everyone who met him. When he first arrived at the Georgetown Hospital ER, he was bleeding so badly internally that he drifted in and out of consciousness. Half his blood had to be replaced by transfusions. Yet once when he briefly regained consciousness, he noticed a nurse holding his hand and joked, "Does Nancy [his wife] know about us?"

Shortly after that, he was taken into surgery to remove a bullet that had stopped an mere inch from his heart. His doctors were worried and tense. None wanted to be known as the one whose mistake killed a President. To ease their tension, Reagan quipped that he hoped they all were Republicans, to which the head surgeon replied something like, "Today, Mr. President, we're all Republicans."

With President Reagan, everyone who cared for him felt his interest in them. While in the hospital recovering, he spent his nights joking with nurses. It's easy to see why they adored a patient who gave them so much attention.

You can do the same. As a teen girl, you can be incredibly infuriating or wonderfully charming. (Just ask your mother.) The choice is yours, so pick the latter. Show your appreciation and demonstrate an interest in those caring for you. Take difficult situations with humor, remembering that it's always safe to make jokes about yourself. If something unpleasant happens, laugh about it rather than throwing a snit or sulking. A good sense of humor is always appealing.

Finally, don't forget to care for the patients around you. Your nurses will notice and appreciate that too. At one point, one of our rooms had so many girls with mental issues, a nurse referred to it as a "psychiatric ward." Yet one girl transformed everything with her interest in the other girls. Even more surprising, she was someone you might think would have the worst problems of all.

Cheryl was about fifteen, with warm and caring eyes. She'd been so badly abused as a baby, one nurse told me that she still had scars from where cigarettes had been snuffed out. Even worse, one of her legs had been so badly broken, it was shorter than the other, causing her to walk with a limp. She only escaped those horrors because a kind and loving couple adopted her.

That short leg brought her into our care. We had a surgery just for her. On the first visit, our surgeons would stop the growth in her longer leg. Then a year or so later, when the shorter leg reached that same length, they'd stop the growth in it. Cheryl would end up a little shorter, but she'd have two legs the same length and a normal walk. That's good.

I still have a picture of her in a wheelchair made when I took her and her mother down to go home. As I did, I told myself that, if I'd been a boy of sixteen, she'd be getting my boyish attention. She was that special. You could do worse than be like her.

You might also read books for inspiration. If you like romances, particularly true-life ones, try *A Severe Mercy* by Sheldon Vanauken. The book is about his much-loved wife, Davy. At one point in her illness, it became clear that she would die so, as he put it, she began to say, "farewell to the wind and sky, watching it all go and fade away, die—and thanking God. And yet she was human, heartbreakingly human, and she did not want to die." He continues:

> She obediently did everything the doctors and the nurses told her to do: everything except to stay in her bed when someone else was in need. Over and over again, she was discovered out of bed in the night, sitting beside some other patient who was suffering, soothing her, holding her hand, praying for her.... Later I would get dozens of letters, some almost illiterate, from people who had been in the hospital with her, saying that she had helped and sustained them. One said she was like an angel of God.

> The nurses loved her and the hospital servants, too. She enlisted my help to make a grand medal, "for faithful service" for one of the black maids, who wore it proudly. Many of the nurses were praying for her.... It is simply true, without exaggeration, to say that she was a tower of strength to everyone.... Love shone forth from her, and love not only begets love, it transmits strength.

Always remember that many of those who enter medicine and nursing are caring people. They wouldn't have chosen the work if they weren't. But the sheer burden of it all, emotionally and physically, often overcomes them. On top of that, hospitals are filled to the brim with suffering and tragedy. The staff, overwhelmed by their work and surrounded by so much pain, often feel they must wall out that sadness out to cope. Treating them as special breaks down those walls. Being funny and showing concern for other patients also helps. You become special. They'll notice you, care for you, and protect you in the tough times.

That's my magic tip, and it's simple. Like Binky, be a joy to those caring for you. Be their favorite patient and they'll look out for you.

NOTES

www.ingramcontent.com/pod-product-compliance
Lightning Source LLC
Chambersburg PA
CBHW020155200326
41521CB00006B/371